Palliative and End of Life Care in Nursing

Transforming Nursing Practice series

Transforming Nursing Practice is the first series of books designed to help students meet the requirements of the NMC Standards and Essential Skills Clusters for degree programmes. Each book addresses a core topic, and together they cover the generic knowledge required for all fields of practice.

Core knowledge titles

Series editor: Professor Shirley Bach, Head of the School of Health Sciences at the University of Brighton

Acute and Critical Care in Adult Nursing	ISBN 978 0 85725 842 7
Becoming a Registered Nurse: Making the Transition to Practice	ISBN 978 0 85725 931 8
Caring for Older People in Nursing	ISBN 978 1 44626 763 9
Communication and Interpersonal Skills in Nursing (2nd edn)	ISBN 978 0 85725 449 8
Contexts of Contemporary Nursing (2nd edn)	ISBN 978 1 84445 374 0
Dementia Care in Nursing	ISBN 978 0 85725 873 1
Getting into Nursing	ISBN 978 0 85725 895 3
Health Promotion and Public Health for Nursing Students (2nd edn)	ISBN 978 1 44627 503 0
Introduction to Medicines Management in Nursing	ISBN 978 1 84445 845 5
Law and Professional Issues in Nursing (3rd edn)	ISBN 978 1 44626 858 2
Leadership, Management and Team Working in Nursing	ISBN 978 0 85725 453 5
Learning Skills for Nursing Students	ISBN 978 1 84445 376 4
Medicines Management in Adult Nursing	ISBN 978 1 84445 842 4
Medicines Management in Children's Nursing	ISBN 978 1 84445 470 9
Nursing Adults with Long Term Conditions	ISBN 978 0 85725 441 2
Nursing and Collaborative Practice (2nd edn)	ISBN 978 1 84445 373 3
Nursing and Mental Health Care	ISBN 978 1 84445 467 9
Nursing in Partnership with Patients and Carers:	ISBN 978 0 85725 307 1
Passing Calculations Tests for Nursing Students (2nd edn)	ISBN 978 1 44625 642 8
Palliative and End of Life Care in Nursing	ISBN 978 1 44627 092 9
Patient and Carer Participation in Nursing	ISBN 978 0 85725 307 1
Patient Assessment and Care Planning in Nursing	ISBN 978 0 85725 858 8
Patient Safety and Managing Risk in Nursing	ISBN 978 1 44626 688 5
Psychology and Sociology in Nursing	ISBN 978 0 85725 836 6
Safeguarding Adults in Nursing Practice	ISBN 978 1 44625 638 1
Successful Practice Learning for Nursing Students (2nd edn)	ISBN 978 0 85725 315 6
Using Health Policy in Nursing	ISBN 978 1 44625 646 6
What is Nursing? Exploring Theory and Practice (3rd edn)	ISBN 978 0 85725 975 2

Personal and professional learning skills titles

Series editors: Dr Mooi Standing, Independent Academic Consultant (UK and International) & Accredited NMC Reviewer and Professor Shirley Bach, Head of the School of Health Sciences at the University of Brighton

Clinical Judgement and Decision Making in Nursing (2nd edn)	ISBN 978 1 44628 281 6
Critical Thinking and Writing for Nursing Students (2nd edn)	ISBN 978 1 44625 644 2
Evidence-based Practice in Nursing (2nd edn)	ISBN 978 1 44627 090 5
Information Skills for Nursing Students	ISBN 978 1 84445 381 8
Reflective Practice in Nursing (2nd edn)	ISBN 978 1 44627 085 1
Succeeding in Essays, Exams & OSCEs for Nursing Students	ISBN 978 0 85725 827 4
Succeeding in Literature Reviews and Research Project Plans for Nursing Students (2nd edn)	ISBN 978 1 44628 283 0
Successful Professional Portfolios for Nursing Students	ISBN 978 0 85725 457 3
Understanding Research for Nursing Students (2nd edn)	ISBN 978 1 44626 761 5

Mental health nursing titles

Series editors: Sandra Walker, Senior Teaching Fellow in Mental Health in the Faculty of Health Sciences, University of Southampton and Professor Shirley Bach, Head of the School of Health Sciences at the University of Brighton

Assessment and Decision Making in Mental Health Nursing	ISBN 978 1 44626 820 9
Engagement and Therapeutic Communication in Mental Health Nursing	ISBN 978 1 44627 480 4
Medicines Management in Mental Health Nursing	ISBN 978 0 85725 049 0
Mental Health Law in Nursing	ISBN 978 0 85725 761 1

You can find more information on each of these titles and our other learning resources at www.sagepub.co.uk. Many of these titles are also available in various e-book formats; please visit our website for more information.

Palliative and End of Life Care in Nursing

Jane Nicol and Brian Nyatanga

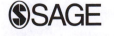

Los Angeles | London | New Delhi
Singapore | Washington DC

CUYAHOGA COMMUNITY COLLEGE
EASTERN CAMPUS LIBRARY

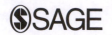

Learning Matters
An imprint of SAGE Publications Ltd
1 Oliver's Yard
55 City Road
London EC1Y 1SP

SAGE Publications Inc.
2455 Teller Road
Thousand Oaks, California 91320

SAGE Publications India Pvt Ltd
B 1/I 1 Mohan Cooperative Industrial Area
Mathura Road
New Delhi 110 044

SAGE Publications Asia-Pacific Pte Ltd
3 Church Street
#10-04 Samsung Hub
Singapore 049483

Editor: Alex Clabburn
Development editor: Caroline Sheldrick
Production controller: Chris Marke
Project management: Swales & Willis Ltd, Exeter, Devon
Marketing manager: Tamara Navaratnam
Cover design: Wendy Scott
Typeset by: C&M Digitals (P) Ltd, Chennai, India
Printed by: Henry Ling Limited at The Dorset Press, Dorchester, DT1 1HD

© Jane Nicol and Brian Nyatanga 2014

First published 2014

Library of Congress Control Number: 2014935438

British Library Cataloguing in Publication Data

A catalogue record for this book is available from the British Library

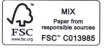

ISBN 978-1-4462-7091-2
ISBN 978-1-4462-7092-9 (pbk)

Dedication

To Priscilla for all the patience, love and supportive smiles given over the years.

To Pamela Lou, Nev and Lewin for keeping me in your youthful world.

To my mother at 103 years old: I salute your greatness and positive guidance always.

To special partners and colleagues for willingness to share experiences unconditionally.

To the late Nelson Mandela for sharing a unique moral compass not only for South Africa but for the whole world to follow.

Brian Nyatanga

Contents

About the authors

Editors

Jane Nicol is a registered nurse and Senior Lecturer at the Institute of Health and Society, Nursing, Midwifery and Paramedic Science, University of Worcester. During her career she has worked across a range of clinical settings in both primary and secondary care, enabling her to develop a broad knowledge and skill base. Jane currently teaches on both the pre-registration nursing programme and the BSc(Hons) international programme focusing on the care and management of long-term conditions and palliative and end of life care. Jane has written previously for the Learning Matters series on long-term conditions management.

Dr Brian Nyatanga is Senior Lecturer at the Institute of Health and Society, Applied Professional Studies, and Lead for The Centre for Palliative Care, which he recently developed jointly with a local hospice. He teaches palliative care and research methods across the university programmes and to international students in the UK and abroad. Brian is aware of the emotional demands of caring for people at the end of life and believes in structured social support for practitioners. His doctoral research thesis investigated death anxiety and burnout among palliative nurses. He is well published, with over 25 years of clinical and educational experience in palliative care.

Contributors

Jean Fisher is Head of Education at St Michael's Hospice, Hereford. Jean trained as a general nurse in Salisbury, Wiltshire, qualifying in 1979. Following a passion for plastic surgery and burns nursing she worked as both a staff nurse and ward sister in this speciality, acquiring post-registration qualifications in both this sphere and orthopaedics. Concerned about the lack of knowledge and skills evident in relation to caring for the dying and bereaved, Jean's interest and enthusiasm for palliative care grew. She first became involved in palliative care in 1984, when she was appointed as a ward sister in a new hospice. Since then Jean has been immersed in palliative and end of life care. She now combines education and management with some clinical activities within her current role.

Hazel Luckhurst is Senior Lecturer at the Institute of Health and Society, Nursing, Midwifery and Paramedic Science, University of Worcester. Her areas of expertise include critical care, leadership and problem-based learning. Hazel has extensive experience in critical care subspecialties such as cardiothoracic, trauma and general and neurological intensive care both in the UK and overseas. In addition Hazel has direct bedside clinical experience supporting patients at the end of life. Hazel has led diploma and degree critical care modules and teaches across nursing programmes which address the changing nature of professional health care.

Sherri Ogston-Tuck is Senior Lecturer at the Institute of Health and Society, Nursing, Midwifery and Paramedic Science, University of Worcester. Her clinical background is in acute adult nursing with an emphasis in law and ethics, pain and medicines management. Sherri undertook her nurse education and training in Canada; this was followed by clinical nursing experiences in emergency and acute adult care in the UK. Sherri has worked in an academic role for over a decade and has a range of publications to her name. Sherri's interest in law and ethics in nursing practice has developed as a result of the emerging role and responsibilities of the nurse, the complexities of the human condition and decision making in health care today. Sherri's Chapter 6 is dedicated to Ian, a colleague and dear friend, who experienced kindness and respect from compassionate health care professionals in his end of life care.

Dr Helen Taylor is Senior Lecturer at the Institute of Health and Society, Applied Professional Studies, University of Worcester. She is a Programme Lead and Senior Lecturer in Health Law at the University of Worcester. She has a PhD in Health Psychology, is a barrister-at-law (non-practising) and has a long-standing research and academic interest, together with a range of publications focusing on the promotion of an individual's right to autonomy, dignity and respect.

Foreword

The bringing together in this book of palliative care nursing, which is relevant to patients at all stages of illness and disease, and end of life care was a deliberate intention to demonstrate the interdependency that both forms of care have with each other. As the editors Jane Nicol and Brian Nyatanga suggest, the sometimes long journey from diagnosis to the end of life requires complex and personalised care and this excellent book provides a comprehensive resource for all aspects of this important aspect of nursing. The book is enriched by contributions from Jean Fisher, Hazel Luckhurst, Sherri Ogston-Tuck and Helen Taylor who are experienced experts and academics.

Beginning with discussions on determining the scope of holistic palliative care that is conveyed, not only to patients, but to their family and those important to them, the book continues by exploring the essential features of communicating with dying patients and their family or carers.

It is impossible not to acknowledge that loss, in its many forms associated with illness whether long term or sudden, dying and death are emotive subjects and can generate a deep sense of hurt and grief. The authors explore these feelings sensitively and professionally through analysis and theoretical models which will help the reader support and guide patients and their families or carers through the labyrinth of these powerful emotions.

The multicultural nature of the UK population constitutes the fabric of our modern society and the nurse's role in palliative and end of life care requires a sensitivity and understanding of different cultural mores. In this book the concepts underpinning culture and the need to be culturally aware and competent to care for patients from different cultural backgrounds is a crucial component and thoughtfully explored.

Dealing with death in any setting is distressing, and the authors take a deeper look at this in a critical care setting where the death significantly contradicts the main purpose of such a unit which is focussed on sustaining life at all costs. This delicate situation is explored in-depth and is a unique feature, distinguishing this text from others in the field.

Ethical considerations and dilemmas are ever present in caring and in particular at the end of life phase. In the final chapters insights into these dilemmas and legal aspects of care are explored using case studies and practical case analysis to assist the reader in untangling this complex moral and ethical topic.

In this book, the Transforming Nursing Practice series has again provided a detailed and comprehensive guide into a fundamental element of nursing care. The book offers a thoughtful and in-depth source of information, theory and research for nursing students or qualified nurses who wish to review their skills and knowledge in a topic that is ever present in our work.

Professor Shirley Bach
Series Editor

Acknowledgements

In producing this book, there were challenges of time, work and social events to balance along the way. We are grateful for the help and support from different people, and in particular the University of Worcester for affording us scholarly leave to write this book. A special thank you must go to all the chapter contributors. Your contribution and willingness to share will inspire everyone who cares to read this book.

The publisher and authors wish to thank the following for permission to reproduce copyright material:

John Wiley and Sons for the figure Trajectories of dying (Figure 2.1) which first appeared in June R. Lunney, Joanne Lynn and Christopher Hogan, 'Profiles of Older Medicare Decedents', *Journal of the American Geriatrics Society*, 50 (6): 1108–1112.

Mark Allan Publishing for an adapted version of the ASSET model (Figure 2.2) from Ellis, H.K. and Narayanasamya, A. (2009) An investigation into the role of spirituality in nursing, *British Journal of Nursing*, 18 (14): 886–890.

Introduction

About this book

The main aim of the book is to discuss some of the key aspects of palliative and end of life care in a simple way that helps understanding. This book is written and edited by experts in the field of palliative and end of life care, and offers the reader a gentle introduction to one of the most complex and sensitive areas of health care practice. It is written in the main for those entering health care professions, like student nurses, student doctors and allied health professionals, who wish to develop their understanding in palliative and end of life care. It is also envisaged that more experienced health care professionals can use this book as a refresher and aide when teaching other members of staff.

Why *Palliative and End of Life Care*?

The title of the book recognises two key facets omnipresent in this field of care: palliative and end of life care. There is recognition of the sometimes long journey from diagnosis to death which characterises palliative care, and the endpoint/final phase of life before physical death (end of life). This can bring about complex emotions and reactions. Palliative and end of life care requires a comprehensive supportive approach by health care professionals to ensure all those in need are helped, cared for and supported in order to adjust to impending death and beyond.

Book structure

The book comprises eight chapters, each focusing on an important aspect of palliative care. Although the book can be read by dipping in and out of chapters, it is recommended that Chapter 1 is read first. This chapter sets the scene, discussing some of the philosophical positions encountered in life, living, dying and death. It is suggested that an appreciation of some of this philosophical discourse is needed before fully understanding the delivery and practice of palliative and end of life care. Chapter 2 discusses holistic palliative care that is delivered, not only to patients, but to their family and those important to them. Such care depends on accurate assessment that identifies patients' needs, wishes and aspirations, even at this final stage in their life. Chapter 3 focuses on the most important, and yet difficult, aspect of care, communicating with a dying patient and his or her family/carers. A number of skills that facilitate effective communication are discussed while potential barriers are also highlighted. Chapter 4 acknowledges that dying and death provoke a sense of loss which is followed by grief which needs to be managed throughout bereavement. This chapter uses some well-known theories and models of loss, grief and bereavement to help the reader to understand how, and why, patients and families may react to death and dying. Chapter 5 recognises the multicultural nature of the UK population, and indeed most countries, and therefore discusses the ideas of culture, culture modifications and the need to be culturally competent to care for patients from different cultural backgrounds. Chapter 6 discusses the ethical considerations and dilemmas present in caring and in particular at the end of life phase. This chapter offers some insights which tend to overlap or link with legal aspects, which are the subject of Chapter 8. Chapter 7 addresses delivering palliative care and end of life care in an intensive care unit. This environment is rarely seen as palliative care and yet a number of people die here each year. Discussing palliative care in an intensive care unit, it serves to illustrate further what Chapter 1 discussed – that the philosophy of palliative care can be practised anywhere as long as someone is dying.

Chapter 8 is the final chapter and gives a series of legal cases as a way of demonstrating the complexity of some of the deliberations lawyers and judges go through and the decisions they make. It is clear that there is a clear distinction between legal and professional positions when caring for other people, and carers in palliative care need to be aware of these.

Requirements for the NMC Standards for Pre-registration Nursing Education and the Essential Skills Clusters

The Nursing and Midwifery Council (NMC) has established standards of competence to be met by applicants to different parts of the register, and these are the standards it considers necessary for safe and effective practice. In addition to the competencies, the NMC has set out specific skills that nursing students must be able to perform at various points of an education programme. These are known as Essential Skills Clusters (ESCs). This book is structured so that it will help you to understand and meet the competencies and ESCs required for entry to the NMC register. The relevant competencies and ESCs are presented at the start of each chapter so that you can clearly see which ones the chapter addresses. There are *generic standards* that all nursing students irrespective of their field must achieve, and *field-specific standards* relating to each field of nursing – mental health, children's, learning disability and adult nursing. Most chapters have generic standards, and occasionally field-specific ones are included.

This book includes the latest standards for 2010 onwards, taken from *Standards for Pre-registration Nursing Education* (NMC 2010).

Learning features

Throughout the book you will find activities in the text that will help you to make sense of, and learn about, the material being presented by the authors.

Some activities ask you to reflect on aspects of practice, or your experience of it, or the people or situations you encounter. *Reflection* is an essential skill in nursing, and it helps you to understand the world around you and often to identify how things might be improved. Other activities will help you develop key skills, such as your ability to *think critically* about a topic in order to challenge received wisdom, or your ability to *research a topic and find appropriate information and evidence*, and to be able to make decisions using that evidence in situations that are often difficult and time-pressured. Finally, communication and working as part of a team are core to all nursing practice, and some activities will ask you to carry out *group activities* or think about your *communication skills* to help develop these.

All the activities require you to take a break from reading the text, think through the issues presented and carry out some independent study, possibly using the internet. Where appropriate, there are sample answers presented at the end of each chapter, and these will help you to understand more fully your own reflections and independent study. Remember, academic study will always require independent work; attending lectures will never be enough to be successful on your programme, and these activities will help to deepen your knowledge and understanding of the issues under scrutiny and give you practice at working on your own.

You might want to think about completing these activities as part of your personal development plan (PDP) or portfolio. After completing the activity write it up in your PDP or portfolio in a section devoted to that particular skill, then look back over time to see how far you are developing. You can also do more of the activities for a key skill in which you have identified a weakness, which will help build your skill and confidence in this area.

Chapter 1
The idea of life, living, dying and death

Brian Nyatanga

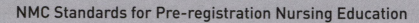

NMC Standards for Pre-registration Nursing Education

This chapter will address the following competencies:

Domain 1: Professional values
2. All nurses must practise in a holistic, non-judgemental, caring and sensitive manner that avoids assumptions, supports social inclusion; recognises and respects individual choice; and acknowledges diversity. Where necessary, they must challenge inequality, discrimination and exclusion from access to care.

Domain 2: Communication and interpersonal skills
1. All nurses must build partnerships and therapeutic relationships through effective and non-discriminatory communication. They must take account of individual differences, capabilities and needs.

Domain 3: Nursing practice and decision making
4. All nurses must ascertain and respond to the physical, social and psychological needs of people, groups and communities. They must then plan, deliver and evaluate safe, competent, person-centred care in partnership with them, paying special attention to changing health needs during different life stages, including progressive illness and death, loss and bereavement.

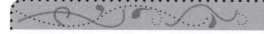

NMC Essential Skills Clusters

This chapter will address the following:

Essential skills cluster: care, compassion and communication
3. People can trust the newly registered graduate nurse to respect them as individuals and strive to help them preserve their dignity at all times.
First progression point
1. Demonstrate respect for diversity and individual preference, valuing differences, regardless of personal view.

Entry to the register
4. Acts professionally to ensure that personal judgements, prejudices, values, attitudes and beliefs do not compromise care.

Chapter aims

After reading this chapter, you will be able to:

- understand the connection between living and dying and how this can improve care for patients receiving palliative and end of life care;
- appreciate why most people continue to fear death and how you can support patients to achieve an individualised death;
- appreciate the role euphemisms play in 'softening' the reality of death and the impact this can have on patients and the bereaved;
- understand what palliative and end of life care are and their underlying ethos;
- explore the practice of palliative and end of life care provision and its impact on quality of life;
- appreciate the importance of dying in your own home and use this information to support patient-centred palliative and end of life care.

Introduction

I am not afraid of death, I just don't want to be there when it happens.
(Woody Allen)

This quote highlights the paradox of how the human mind perceives life and death. It recognises the tension between what we know and what we don't know and the fears that are inherent in both. The aim of this chapter is to allow you to explore this, and similar conflicting ideas surrounding life and death, and to use this knowledge to enable you to provide person-centred care for patients receiving palliative and end of life care. The quote also identifies some philosophical areas about living and dying, and how these two notions connect with each other. It is no secret that most people tend to fear death even though they all know it will happen to them at some point in their life. This chapter will discuss and offer arguments as to why this remains the case. The discussion will also look at how death has remained a taboo topic throughout Western societies. The taboo nature of death can be explained by the use of euphemisms around the aspects of death and dying. This chapter will ask you to think through why euphemisms still have a place in our language and whether their use is beneficial, or a hindrance, to our attempts to talk openly about death. It is important that you, and other health care professionals, develop the knowledge and skills necessary to feel confident to care for patients who are at the end of their life (palliative care). In order to do this, you will need to understand the principles that govern the practice of palliative care. The ethos which underpins the delivery of palliative care is central to offering the best care possible to all patients.

It is true that patients now die in different places, including hospices, hospitals and nursing homes, and most prefer to die in their own home. Why dying in the home is preferred and what could be driving or influencing these decisions will also be discussed. What is important in all aspects of the care and support you offer to patients is that it will improve or enhance their quality of life. Quality of life aims to ensure a dignified and unique death for each patient. The importance of achieving a dignified death is manifold. One important aspect is that it helps relatives as they go through their bereavement.

The connection between living and dying

Plants and animals are living things, whereas objects are not: they exist, but are not alive. It is generally thought that only animals (including humans) have consciousness. You are living in the sense that you are breathing, your heart is pumping blood around your body and your mind is either conscious or unconscious. People are considered to be dying when something threatens their prospect of living, such as terminal illness, but also when they are ageing. When you look closely at this, it is impossible to talk about death without considering life as the two are part of a continuum. In addition, life itself is one of those concepts that remains unclearly defined. When does life (living) stop in order for dying to start? Most people would agree that life (living) is the beginning of death (dying), which in turn signals the end of life. Looking at life and death in this way gives one example of how language can create uncertainty (linguistic ambiguity) due to lack of clarity in what is meant by such expressions. The other point to consider is that, although we know death is a certainty, we rarely talk openly about it and are therefore still fearful of it.

Activity 1.1   *Reflection*

This activity is to allow you time to reflect on how you view life and death and to think about when both life and death start.

When people are born we like to think that this is when their living starts.

Write down your thoughts about this and say whether you agree with such thinking. Now write down when you think dying starts.

Brief answers to all activities are given at the end of the chapter, unless otherwise indicated. This activity is based on your own observations, so there is no outline answer given.

Your reflections in Activity 1.1 will be unique to you and this will be the same for your patients. However, there are legal positions about when life starts. In the UK it is when a pregnancy is 22 weeks and in the USA it is 20 weeks. The legal positions are not going to be discussed here; the important point for you to think about is whether we can separate living from dying. Nyatanga and Nyatanga (2011) suggest that these two things tend to happen at the same time. The argument they make is that, as you grow from an infant to an adult (living), you are also gradually dying. You could argue that what we call living is the same as what we call dying because these two aspects/processes happen at the same time. If you accept this, you can go on to suggest that life is to do with this process (living/dying) and death is in a simplistic way the end of this process.

Most people enjoy their youth and growing up; not many people will consciously think about their dying at the same time. Even people who become ill in their youth rarely consider that they might die. This may in some way explain the absolute horror we feel when a child or young adult dies; our minds are not always prepared for a young person's death.

This may not be the case in other parts of the world; we see images of death in developing countries due to famine, war or drought which involve children and young adults. We can, wrongly, come to accept that as part of the harsh reality of their life. However the recent shooting of young children at a primary school in the USA can seem more shocking and unexpected as these deaths took place in a developed country. This illustrates how living, dying and death may be perceived differently in these countries. Death in developing countries is not always preventable and may be viewed as part of everyday life, whereas in the UK we have the means of postponing death. People living in Western nations might not encounter death in their family until they are in their sixties. The different experiences we have of living and dying shape our perception of death. The point to remember is that, although death may be the same with regard to how we define it, our perception of it will differ according to individual experiences. Equally, the meaning of death will differ depending on individual experiences and in some cases beliefs that we hold about life.

Activity 1.2   *Reflection*

Reflect on your own perception of death, and then respond to the following points:

- What do you think death is? Write down your thoughts.
- Make a note on aspects of your life that have made you view death in this way, such as religious beliefs.
- How might your perception of death influence the way you care for patients at the end of their life?

The following part of this activity is optional. If it brings back painful emotional memories or reactions, please feel free not to do it.

- Cast your mind back to the very first time you witnessed a human death; write down how old you were at the time. Describe how you think the whole experience affected you and influenced how you feel about death now. Of course, the experience will also depend on who it was that died (whether the person was close to you or not), how the individual died and how old this person was at the time.

As this activity is based on your own observations, there is no outline answer at the end of this chapter.

You might have found Activity 1.2 quite difficult to complete as there is a lack of tangible evidence about what death is really like. Nobody has come back from the dead to tell us about their own experience of death. In addition our perceptions are formed from a range of experiences during our day-to-day life and vary from person to person. It is likely that you have arrived at your perception of death using the experiences of your own life so far. Your perceptions are formed by the things you encounter as you grow up, therefore we can conclude that people are not born with a perception of death. If you agree that people are not born with a perception of death, it follows that these perceptions are learned and are formed by each person as they go through life. You learn things which guide your thinking and behaviour and at the same time you can unlearn things or learn new things that can change your original way of thinking and behaving.

What this suggests is that you and your patients are most likely to have different perceptions of death, and therefore of what death is. Therefore if you are going to help patients with their own dying, you need to understand what death means for them. To do this you need to understand how the patient's history (previous experiences of death) might have shaped the way he or she views death now. Further information about this can be found in Chapter 4: Exploring loss, grief and bereavement.

Death as taboo

To delight in talking about death, particularly the prospect of one's own death, is, in Western society, often considered morbid. As a consequence the topic of death and dying has become a taboo subject culminating in people fearing death (Twycross 2003; Nyatanga and Nyatanga 2011). Currently in the UK, not many children are involved in the death of a family member, which means that the first time that you encounter death might be when you come into nursing. Talking openly about death has the potential to make it easier to deal with. It becomes a familiar topic to most people, including children, as they grow up. Recognising why people fear death and how this relates to you and your patients will help you to begin to have open conversations with patients and their families, supporting them to face the reality of their situation.

Fear of death

Most people remain fearful of death and with that we have to argue also that people worry about life. For example, if life were perfect and enjoyable, then most people would like to hold on to it and continue living. Human beings will resist death at any cost; they might pay large sums of money or invest time and resources to preserve life. This would not be the case if life was full of problems, complications and was purposeless. There is an inevitable link between life and death in that life with its perpetual problems and complications may make us prefer death as a way of finding an exit point (death-oriented). The opposite is also true: people who love life immensely (life-oriented) will most certainly be fearful of death, because it takes away the very essence of living which they hold dear. Whichever way we look at this we are in fact fearful of death and worried about life. The main difference is that with life you have a choice of what to do, but you rarely have a choice about death and how it comes. This apparent helplessness may explain why most people continue to fear death. In most situations where helplessness is experienced many things happen: the two main ones are loss of control and loss of independence. Dying patients often explain how their disease has made them helpless and unable to fulfil their 'duties' as father, mother, brother, sister or any one of the roles they used to have. It is the loss of these roles and duties that emphasises loss of control and independence for that person. This in turn can promote fear of the future and fear of death.

Activity 1.3   *Reflection*

Take the time to reflect on what it is about death that makes you fear it. If you do not fear death, reflect on why this is and why some people may fear death. You may wish to discuss this with colleagues or friends.

As this activity is based on your own observations, there is no outline answer at the end of this chapter.

In Activity 1.3 you may have begun your reflection by asking yourself further questions about your fear of death. For example:

- Why is it that people fear death despite the fact that it is a certainty for each and every one of us?
- Even without knowing what lies beyond death (the unknown), why are people still fearful of death?
- Is it at all possible that the unknown itself could be something quite pleasant?

These are not easy questions to answer and even philosophers and psychologists have failed to reach unanimous agreement. The philosopher Plato (427–347 BC) presented key points from Socrates' argument about fearing death thus:

To fear death, gentlemen, is no other than to think oneself wise when one is not, to think one knows what one does not know. No one knows whether death may not be the greatest of all blessings for man, yet men fear it as if they knew that it is the greatest of evils. And surely it is the most blameworthy ignorance to believe that one knows what one does not know.

Although Socrates was making a philosophical and logical argument, even now our minds do not seem to be persuaded to stop fearing death. There may be many ways of explaining why this remains the case. Some people fear death because it interrupts their life. Death can interrupt a young life, middle-aged life or old life, male or female, rich or poor. Death does not distinguish between black and white, able-bodied or disabled, religious or agnostic and even good and bad people; this makes it indiscriminate and unpredictable (Nyatanga and Nyatanga 2011). If death is not upon us, it is happening elsewhere with someone we know. The media and newspapers are constantly reminding us of death and by extension emphasising how temporary our own life is. This constant reminder makes people more anxious about their life ending and therefore makes them worry more about their death (death anxiety) and that of those most near and dear to us.

The indiscriminate nature of death makes it hard for the human mind to understand how death 'operates'. In life we tend to understand most things, but death is elusive and less predictable. When you look at death in this way, you can begin to see how the irrefutable fact of death creates fear for many people. Medical advances and research have tried to change the course of death, or even avoid it altogether, without success.

Ideas from biology (Brown 2008) give clear guidance that, as one generation grows old, it gives room (through death) for the next one and thereby benefits the species. Biological ideas can only be used to a certain point. The reality of our life is that we spend it growing up well and creating unique identities, working hard, educating ourselves, forming relationships, having desires and gathering possessions – only to be denied all these things by ageing and death.

Our patients are no different from us and they too can experience these realities. Encouraging them to focus on positive experiences could play an important role when we care for dying patients.

Case study

Johnny

Johnny is 53 years old; he was diagnosed with terminal small cell lung cancer six months ago. He lives with his wife Sandra in a semidetached three-bedroom house; they have two children, Megan and James, aged 28 and 25. Megan and James live locally, Megan with her husband; they are expecting their first child in three months. James lives in a shared house with two friends. Johnny has been a member of the local Hell's Angels since he was 18. He met Sandra when he was 23 at a Hell's Angels meeting. They both ride motorbikes and spend most of their time out travelling and touring on their bikes.

Until this diagnosis Johnny was fairly fit, though he has smoked since he was 17. He has tried to give up but without success; the longest period of time he stopped for was eight months. Six months ago Johnny noticed that he was becoming breathless and had a cough. He first noticed this at work when pushing the motorbikes (he worked at a local motorbike garage). Shortly after this he developed a wheeze. Sandra was the first to notice this and, after much prompting, Johnny visited his GP. A chest X-ray revealed multiple tumours in both lungs, and a CT scan confirmed liver metastasis. Due to the extent of his disease surgical excision was not possible; Johnny was offered a course of radiotherapy and chemotherapy. Following this there was an initial improvement in his main symptoms of cough and dyspnoea; however these have worsened again. In addition to this Johnny is now fatigued. Johnny and his family are aware of his poor prognosis and that he may only have months left to live; his main aim is to be alive for the birth of his first grandchild.

Johnny remains fiercely independent; he is reluctant to allow Sandra to help him. It can sometimes take him most of the day to get up, washed and dressed. Sandra is keen to be involved in caring for Johnny; however she knows not to push this. Sandra would like to begin to discuss what care Johnny might need in the future. At the moment Sandra continues to work as a teaching assistant at a local high school; she enjoys this as it gives her a focus outside home. Both Megan and James visit their mum and dad daily. Megan is still working as a dental assistant and James works as a CAD engineer for a local manufacturing company.

Johnny has reluctantly stopped riding his motorbike, though his Hell's Angels friends visit and take him out. This is not the same as riding his own bike but Johnny looks forward to these visits and the feeling of being free when on the bike. Both Johnny and Sandra have a tremendous feeling of support from the camaraderie of the Hell's Angels; Sandra knows that if she needs anything, she only has to ask.

The following activity asks you to consider the situation of Johnny, from the case study, and attempt to make sense of what you could do to support him and his family.

Activity 1.4   *Critical thinking*

- Consider Johnny's diagnosis, prognosis and the needs/symptoms he is presenting with, and make a note of what you think Johnny's main priority in life is at the moment. You will need to say why you think this is his main priority, and this could be a way of explaining your own judgement of Johnny's situation using your nursing or caring skills.
- How would you help and support Johnny and his family to adjust and cope with his illness? Here you need to think of strategies (psychological) and activities (practical) that you think will help Johnny.

An outline answer is given at the end of this chapter.

The first part of Activity 1.4 may produce individual judgements of Johnny's priorities and you would need to check (confirm) this with Johnny himself when you next assess him. Your judgement of his priority may have been influenced by a number of things, including: previous experience of caring for someone like Johnny, or something you once read about as part of your education. In Activity 1.4 you may have encouraged Johnny to reminisce and reflect on the positive memories in his, and his family's, life. For some patients their reminiscence may be painful, but it is important that you remember that the process itself can ultimately be therapeutic. Therefore you should feel confident to support them when they relate to negative experiences. Further information about supportive communication skills can be accessed in the discussion in Chapter 3. In addition, the real skill is to know how and when to 'lift them out of the emotional dip' and let them focus on the positive experiences again.

It is likely that, although there are perceived benefits to talking about death and dying as a means of reducing fear, most people continue to fear death. As a result death may not always be spoken about openly, making death a taboo. Dying Matters is a UK-based coalition of over 30,000 members which aims to encourage the public, health care professionals and other organisations, such as schools, to discuss death and dying openly (see useful websites section at the end of this chapter for the web link). Their aim is to raise awareness of dying, death and bereavement by providing resources, e.g. information leaflets, about how to start a conversation with someone who is dying. Providing people who are dying with the opportunity to discuss their future allows them to set their affairs in order, make a will and think about funeral arrangements. This, in turn, supports their family and friends when they are bereaved. Another way in which people try to 'distance' themselves from death is to use terms like 'passed away' or 'passed over' instead of 'died'. What you have to ask yourself is whether such words help or hinder our attempts to familiarise ourselves with death.

The role of euphemisms

It is common to hear people using euphemisms when referring to death. It is clear that the use of euphemisms does not change the reality of death but somehow offers false and ritualistic reassurances which often mask the impulse to panic or temptation to escape from it all. The language of euphemisms tends to convey kindness through words society deems acceptable to describe the dead person. This may also suggest a deep-seated fear of facing up to death. Just like the fear of the possibility of having no further existential (living) possibilities, euphemisms express a pervasive fear of the unknown. You may have heard terms such as 'he has been called to rest', 'she has gone to sleep' or 'he is singing with the angels'. You may have seen RIP written on grave stones or sympathy cards. This euphemism suggests the dead person is resting in peace and this is seen as being sensitive and more acceptable than saying the person is dead. The fear of death of self and that of loved ones brings about a pseudo-humbleness (softening the harshness of death) and caring expressed through euphemisms. Nyatanga (2008a) claims that the media and in particular newspaper obituaries seem a rich platform for these death euphemisms. Obituaries are more than cultural rituals. They have a strong social and cultural function for most people (for a more detailed discussion of euphemisms, read Nyatanga 2008a, Chapter 10).

Activity 1.5   *Communication*

This activity asks you to reflect on whether you think euphemisms play a useful role in assisting nurses and health care professionals to face death.

- What terms do you use to avoid saying 'dead' or 'death'?
- How do you think the use of euphemisms helps or hinders the way nurses (and other health care professionals) discuss death with their patient?

As this activity is based on your own observations, there is no outline answer at the end of this chapter.

Using euphemisms for death originated with the belief that to speak the word 'death' was to invite death. A common theory holds that death is a taboo subject in most cultures for precisely this reason. We now know that this is an irrational belief, but we continue to hold on to it. In Activity 1.5 you may have stated that euphemisms help soften the impact of death and therefore are a useful tool which shows our sensitive side of caring. Walsh and Nelson (2003) suggest that to be sensitive is the art of saying the same thing in a different way so that we can lessen the hurt or distress death often causes. It's not what you say, but how you say it that makes a difference to the other person. You may also have written about the negative aspects of using euphemisms, especially when misunderstandings may result. An example might result from nurses or doctors saying to relatives, 'We lost your husband this morning', when what they really mean is, 'Your husband died this morning'. It may be said that one is not dying, but *fading away quickly* because *the end is near. Deceased* is a euphemism for dead and sometimes the *deceased* is said to have *gone to a better place.* This is primarily used among the religious with a concept of an afterlife, or Heaven.

The tendency for nurses to use euphemisms as a defence mechanism against death anxiety most likely begins with their cultural and religious socialisation. For most people, dependence on parents and society as role models has a lot to do with the eventual inauthenticity and self-deception inherent in euphemisms. First, euphemisms serve to soften the impact of death on family, friends, community and society and also reduce the associated fear of death. Second, euphemisms encourage the portrayal of positive perceptions within a death, focusing on the 'good' aspects of the person who has died. The use of euphemisms remains widespread; further information about this can be found in both the further reading and useful websites sections at the end of this chapter.

Many people still find death hard to accept and even harder to talk about openly and honestly. Dying in hospital settings or any institution can present its own challenges as they are not seen as the preferred places for dying by most people.

Preferred place of care: dying at home

There is evidence (Higginson and Sen-Gupta 2000) to suggest that most people would prefer to die in their own home. The question is whether this makes death itself any easier, less feared and more private.

Before the industrial revolution, people died in their own homes surrounded by family and close friends. Aries (1974) made claims that death was very much a private family affair. The suggestion here may be that people saw themselves primarily as part of a family unit and less as individuals, and by extension very much part of a community. Viewing life and death through such a community prism meant that the collective celebration at birth and solidarity in death were important. In this pre-industrial context death was encountered early and we could be right in thinking that many people became familiar with its presence.

Aries claims that the nineteenth century saw a shift of attitudes in favour of *death of the other*. Life and its meaning were now seen through the relationships (personal or intimate) people formed with others. As a result, death was seen as the loss of such relationships. In order for the relationships to develop and flourish, privacy was crucial, if not a prerequisite. Therefore, it followed that any death that took place would no longer be a public event, which means death was no longer being mourned as a loss to the community but a physical separation from a loved one (Nyatanga 2008a).

What followed in the twentieth century was an attitude of *death denied* (Aries 1974). Two things became clear: there were different meanings of death and sense of cultural belonging. Some cultures wanted to continue with private death, whilst others preferred to share their loss with those important to them. It can be argued that relatives who did not have close relations would end up taking their relative to hospital (or institution) for support and company whilst receiving help with symptom management.

Below is an activity that will allow you to reflect upon your own preferences to be cared for and eventually to die. What is important to think about is how much of that decision is entirely yours, and how much is influenced by others, circumstances, cultural and religious values. We know from evidence (see discussion of Thomas (2008) below) that there are many factors to consider when deciding on your preference of place of care. The important point to allude to here is that dying is a process socially engineered by other people, even though there is only one person dying at the time.

Activity 1.6   *Reflection*

Take some time to reflect on the following:

- Where would you like to be cared for (e.g. home, hospital, hospice) and where would you like to be when you die?
- Explain why you have chosen this preference.
- Would your decision be influenced by your family, especially if they did not want you to die in your preferred place of death?
- What might be the impact of where you die on you and your family?

As this activity is based on your own observations, there is no outline answer at the end of this chapter.

The decision of where to be cared for or die is left to the patient to make, although in reality, the patient may not have the full range of choices or permission to choose the option. There are many factors to consider when making a decision of where you want to be cared for and die. For example, whether there is space (that is, beds) in the hospice you prefer, or whether family members also prefer you to die in the family home. Some people may experience difficult and complex symptoms that require hospital/hospice admission for effective management. The home may not have all the medication and equipment needed to control and manage symptoms being experienced.

Research summary

Thomas, C. (2008) Dying: places and preferences. In: Payne, S., Seymour, J. and Ingleton, C. (eds) *Palliative Care Nursing: Principles and Evidence Based Practice*, 2nd edn. Maidenhead: McGraw-Hill, Open University Press.

Thomas (2008) reports on the findings from her qualitative study about preferences in place of death by cancer patients in the UK. In her report, she highlighted some of the factors that made these patients choose their preferred places. Patients' attitudes to death played an important part in the decision. The attitudes were also influenced by patients' previous involvement with death, and where the death took place.

Thomas (2008) also found that if patients knew they would have a sense of dignity in their preferred place of care, this was often the deciding factor in choosing where to die.

Thomas (2008) did not come to any firm conclusions about how previous experiences have an impact on the deaths of the cancer patients she was studying. Having a religious faith or not made little difference in preference of place of death. Other factors, such as availability of services and resources, played a part in the final decision of place of care. At times the reputation of services played a huge part in a patient's decision about place of care. Thomas makes the point that services patients deemed effective in meeting their individual needs during the illness phase may be as appealing as a preferred place of death. For those patients who preferred to die at home, it was critical that they had a willing family to be with them and offer support.

What we do not know from this study is whether we can say anything about the impact of previous experiences of death on one's own death.

For example, if patients had positive previous experiences of death, would this mean they are likely to be positive about their own death? It may be quite difficult to be sure about this, so the only way of understanding the impact of previous experience may be down to our own speculation. For example, we may conclude that if individuals had positive previous experiences, they are likely to view their own death in a favourable way.

The idea of dignity is so important to the patient and yet it is least understood by health care professionals. Dignity is about who that person is and ensuring that the care maintains it and at the same time preserves the person's identity. Patients often find themselves struggling to maintain their dignity in the face of aggressive disease that continually erodes their bodies. For example, patients with fungating and odorous tumours struggle to maintain their dignity. Patients can experience social erosion as they face the end of their life, and nurses and other professionals should be there to support them and restore some of their social networks (Astley-Pepper 2005).

There is a large discrepancy between the number of patients who wish to die at home and the actual number that do so. It could be argued that families play a part in influencing what happens; indeed, you may have recognised this in your reflection in Activity 1.6. The patient is part of a family unit, so it becomes quite important that their preferences are also shared by the whole family. The impact of a relative dying at home can have serious consequences, e.g. a family might sell their home because their dad died there and they felt uncomfortable living in the house afterwards. Another family might not be able to use the room where their mum died and board it off from the rest of the house. When discussing preferred place of death, consequences like these need to be considered. Despite agreeing to support their dad to die at home, the family in the case study on page 10 changed their views after their dad had died. It is impossible to know in advance what might happen; however, the point is that we should be aware of these possibilities and find a way of raising these issues with the family at opportune moments.

The discrepancy in where patients at end of life die and where they want to die tells us that there is more work to be done if we are to meet the needs of dying patients. Some of this work is based in the principles and practice of palliative care. The practice of palliative care is founded in a global philosophy aimed at ensuring that every patient approaching the end of life enjoys an enhanced quality of life.

An overview of the principles and practice of palliative and end of life care

The word 'palliative' can be understood from the English meaning of 'palliate'. The *Compact Oxford English Dictionary* describes 'to palliate' as: *making the symptoms of a disease less severe without curing it* (p731). The main aim is promote comfort by making symptoms less severe. In practice, the idea of palliative care comes from the Greek word *pallium*, which means to cloak. The symptoms presented by patients with life-threatening illness are *cloaked* (Twycross 2003) with interventions aimed at alleviating the discomfort.

Before the principles of palliative care are discussed we should take time to consider when should, and when does, palliative care begin? Activity 1.7 will give you the opportunity to explore this.

Activity 1.7   *Critical thinking*

When do you think palliative care should be introduced to patients diagnosed with life-threatening/limiting disease? In your answer state your reasons for the timing.

To help you answer this activity, refer to the book by R.G. Twycross (2003) (*Introducing Palliative Care*, 4th edn. Oxford: Oxford University Press) and read pages 1–7.

As this activity is based on your own observations, there is no outline answer at the end of this chapter.

As you will have seen, modern thinking suggests that palliative care should start at diagnosis of a life-threatening illness, but other views suggest it should start at a different stage. The original definition offered by the World Health Organization, published in 1990, reflects some of the key points you might have included in Activity 1.7. It states:

> *Palliative care is the active total care of patients with life-limiting disease and their families, by a multi-professional team, when the disease is no longer responsive to curative or life-prolonging treatments.*
> (World Health Organization 1990)

This definition has since been revised in line with new developments and thinking in palliative care to the latest one in 2012, thus:

> *Palliative care is an approach that improves the quality of life of patients and their families facing the problems associated with life-threatening illness, through the prevention and relief of suffering by means of early identification and impeccable assessment and the treatment of pain and other problems, physical, psychological and spiritual.*
>
> (World Health Organization 2012)

These definitions emphasise the fact that palliative care extends across all dimensions of the patient, not just the physical. Patients may have psychological, social, spiritual, emotional and even intellectual needs and palliative care aims to address all of them. This approach of caring for all these different aspects of the patient is referred to as total care and is depicted in Figure 1.1 as the PEPSSI approach (Nyatanga 2008a).

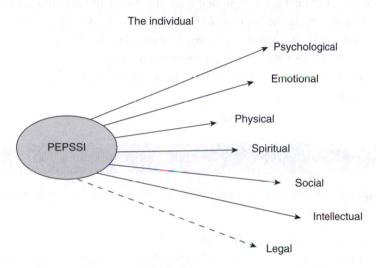

Figure 1.1: The PEPSSI approach to palliative care.

This approach is used in Chapter 2 when discussing holistic care in palliative and end of life care. With recent cases of litigation in health care, some commentators now add 'L' for 'legal' to the PEPSSI approach to indicate the litigious side of health care (this is discussed further in Chapter 8).

Principles of palliative care

The World Health Organization developed eight main guiding principles, listed on page 18. It is important to look at these as guiding principles, because their implementation depends on the health care system of each country, the attitudes towards death commonly held and the availability of medicines such as opioids and the many other resources necessary to care for and support patients receiving palliative care. These principles are prone to flaws, but on the whole they serve to equip health care professionals working with dying patients with the knowledge and skills to help care for their distressing symptoms. Such care would not discriminate against diagnosis, age, ethnicity or sexual orientation.

1. Affirms life and regards dying as a normal process
2. Intends neither to hasten nor postpone death
3. Provides relief from pain and other distressing symptoms
4. Integrates the psychological and spiritual aspects of patient care
5. Offers a support system to help patients live as actively as possible until death
6. Offers a support system to help the family cope during the patient's illness and in their own bereavement
7. Uses a team approach to address the needs of patients and their families, including bereavement counselling, if indicated
8. Will enhance quality of life and may also positively influence the course of illness.

The importance of including a team approach is a reflection of the multiple and complex needs of dying patients, which would be impossible for only nurses or doctors to meet. The composition of a typical palliative care team is discussed below. The idea of a team is that Together Everyone Achieves More (TEAM). This team approach means that the workload and emotional demands of caring for dying patients is shared, thereby protecting each other from excessive stress and even burnout.

Activity 1.8	*Team working*

Palliative and end of life care requires a multidisciplinary team approach. Make a list of all the people you think are part of the multidisciplinary team.

An outline answer is given at the end of this chapter.

Did you include the patient and family/carers in your list in Activity 1.8? In some situations health care professionals can forget that they are there for the patient and his or her needs. The emphasis in palliative and end of life care on holistic person-centred care indicates that, when the team meets to discuss patient needs, the patient is part of the team. In some situations it is not always possible to have the patient present; therefore it is important that the patient's views are represented. This can be done by talking to the patient before the team meeting or inviting family and carers along. In addition processes such as statements of wishes and preferences and advance care planning can be used to ensure a person-centred focus. See the useful websites section at the end of this chapter for further information about these processes.

Since it would be hard to make the patient part of your team every time, having someone (such as a current or previous patient) to represent the views of other patients may solve the problem to some extent. This is the idea of 'user' involvement. This concept can also work in education and training, when we invite participants to come back and be part of our curriculum-planning team for the next education course we deliver for your group or discipline. You would have had experience of current education and can offer suggestions on how to improve it for future courses. The same idea is used with palliative care patients or carers (users) and they often contribute valuable information to the team.

When individuals are healthy, they are part of a family unit and are still part of that unit when they become ill and are dying. Caring for the family as well as the patient recognises this fact. Knowing that the family is being cared for reassures patients, allowing them to feel relaxed enough to concentrate their energies on dealing with their symptoms. In the end, when all the principles are followed and implemented properly, Twycross (2003), Nyatanga (2008a), World Health Organization (2012) and De Souza (2012) all suggest these will enhance the quality of life for the dying patient. By extension the principles will achieve a unique and dignified death for the patient, and one that is witnessed by the family.

Where palliative care takes place

There are many settings, such as hospices, hospitals, nursing homes and the community, where palliative care is delivered (Twycross 2003). While this is true, the key point to remember is that, as a philosophy, palliative care can and should be delivered anywhere there is a patient at the end of life. As we have previously discussed in this chapter, the preferred place of care for many dying patients is their own home. However, it is also recognised that this is not always possible. Therefore palliative care should be delivered in any environment where a patient is dying.

Some environments such as hospices are better equipped to care for palliative care patients than others, therefore it is not surprising that evidence (Thomas 2008; De Souza 2012) tells us that most patients prefer to be cared for and die in hospices. Hospices offer a range of services. For example, patients with complex symptoms can be admitted to an inpatient unit and have their symptoms controlled. The role of palliative and end of life care in a critical care setting is discussed in Chapter 7.

Conclusion

The idea of living, life, dying and death is intricate and therefore it is not easy to see where each aspect starts and the other ends. It looks like dying starts with the start of living, with the focus more on living in early and healthy life. It is beyond doubt that most people know and probably accept (privately) that one day they will die and yet they find it hard to talk openly about their own death. Most people accept that life and living will one day be interrupted by dying and death, therefore you should encourage open discussion about death and dying with patients who are receiving palliative and end of life care. Open dialogue creates opportunities for the patient and family to say goodbye, mend 'bridges', say sorry for mistakes or misunderstandings, write or rewrite wills. The knowledge that patients are dying can spur them to put their own house in order, make that visit to relatives that they have been putting off and make many other important arrangements. Therefore death can be an unexpected bonus and a platform to make final arrangements in this life. However, dying and death can provoke emotions and anticipatory loss, therefore you should provide effective palliative care that offers support and ensures a dignified death.

Good palliative care should be seen as a philosophy that can be delivered in multiple care settings following the patient on the life journey. Places like hospices can be leading examples for good palliative care, and such exemplars of care should be taken into other settings like hospitals, nursing homes and the community. It is important your care is also extended to the patient's family. They too have needs and concerns. The ultimate goal is to achieve a dignified death free from suffering and an enhanced quality of life.

Caring for people who are dying at the end of life is about the quality of the remaining life and not the quantity. The motto from the Nairobi Hospice captures this concept succinctly:

> *Put life into their days, and not days into their life.*
> (The Nairobi Hospice)

Activities: brief outline answers

Activity 1.4: Critical thinking

One important fact for Johnny to realise and appreciate is how to adjust his wishes and hopes to reflect or be in line with the reality of his own illness. Twycross (2003) talks about the need to ensure that patients do not lose hope about their future aspirations. Instead, they should be encouraged and helped to review their hopes and align these with the demands or difficulties of their illness. For example, Johnny feels fatigue and riding his own bike may now be risky, therefore it would be sensible to support Johnny to get a ride with someone else, and still fulfil his hope, albeit differently now.

Activity 1.8: Team working

You may have included the following in your answer to this activity: specialist nurse, medical doctor, occupational therapist, physiotherapist, pharmacist, dietician, speech and language therapist (SaLT), complementary therapist, bereavement support worker, educationalist, researcher, chaplain, family support worker, patient, relatives and informal carers.

Further reading

Gomes, B., Calazani, N. and Higginson, I. (2011) *Local Preferences and Place of Death in Regions Within England 2010.* London: Cicely Saunders International Centre, Kings College.

This report looked at where people prefer to die and ended up dying within the regions of the UK. It is a useful report as it breaks down the preferences by region and therefore gives readers a more specific picture.

Nyatanga, L. and Nyatanga, B. (2011) Death and dying. In: Birchenall, P. and Adams, N. (eds) *The Nursing Companion.* Basingstoke: Palgrave Macmillan, pp179–200.

This chapter outlines a lifespan view of death and dying and how society views, copes with and talks about death. It challenges some rituals and practices found in our society and offers explanations of why death is still a difficult topic to discuss openly. The chapter also offers models to help people in the bereavement phase.

Useful websites

http://www.bored.com/deathslang

This website provides a list of euphemisms people use instead of the words death or dead.

http://dyingmatters.org

This is the website for Dying Matters, a broad based coalition of members whose aim is to change public knowledge and attitudes towards dying, death and bereavement.

http://www.goldstandardsframework.org.uk/advance-care-planning

This website provides you with information about advance care planning, including links to additional sites.

Chapter 2
Holistic patient care in palliative and end of life care

Jane Nicol

NMC Standards for Pre-registration Nursing Education

This chapter will address the following competencies:

Domain 3: Nursing practice and decision making
1. All nurses must use up-to-date knowledge and evidence to assess, plan, deliver and evaluate care, communicate findings, influence change and promote health and best practice. They must make person-centred, evidence-based judgements and decisions, in partnership with others involved in the care process, to ensure high quality care. They must be able to recognise when the complexity of clinical decisions requires specialist knowledge and expertise, and consult or refer accordingly.
3. All nurses must carry out comprehensive, systematic nursing assessments that take account of relevant physical, social, cultural, psychological, spiritual, genetic and environmental factors, in partnership with service users and others through interaction, observation and measurement.
4. All nurses must ascertain and respond to the physical, social and psychological needs of people, groups and communities. They must then plan, deliver and evaluate safe, competent, person-centred care in partnership with them, paying special attention to changing health needs during different life stages, including progressive illness and death, loss and bereavement.

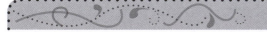

NMC Essential Skills Clusters

This chapter will address the following:

Cluster: Organisational aspects of care
9. People can trust the newly registered graduate nurse to treat them as partners and work with them to make a holistic and systematic assessment of their needs; to develop a personalised plan that is based on mutual understanding and respect for their individual situation promoting health and well-being, minimising risk of harm and promoting their safety at all times.

Second progression point

9. Undertakes the assessment of physical, emotional, psychological, social, cultural and spiritual needs, including risk factors by working with the person and records, shares and responds to clear indicators and signs.

10. With the person and under supervision, plans safe and effective care by recording and sharing information based on the assessment.

Entry to the register

12. In partnership with the person, their carers and their families, makes a holistic, person-centred and systematic assessment of physical, emotional, psychological, social, cultural and spiritual needs, including risk, and together, develops a comprehensive personalised plan of nursing care.

10. People can trust the newly registered graduate nurse to deliver nursing interventions and evaluate their effectiveness against the agreed assessment and care plan.

Second progression point

1. Acts collaboratively with people and their carers enabling and empowering them to take a shared and active role in the delivery and evaluation of nursing interventions.

Entry to the register

6. Provides safe and effective care in partnership with people and their carers within the context of people's ages, conditions and developmental stages.

Chapter aims

After reading this chapter you will be able to:

- consider the concept of holistic care in relation to palliative and end of life care;
- undertake a holistic assessment and use this to plan, implement and evaluate care for those receiving palliative and end of life care;
- apply the principles of effective symptom management to support the care of people requiring palliative and end of life care;
- recognise the role of spiritual care in providing holistic care for those receiving palliative and end of life care.

Introduction

*Sometimes I felt invisible, nurses would walk past, not making eye contact, not seeing me. Don't get me wrong, the treatment I had was great, but . . . the **care** . . . I just wanted someone to look at me, to be aware of me and to recognise who I was, not just a person with cancer.*

(Male, aged 47 with a malignant brain tumour; emphasis added)

Attending to the holistic care needs of patients who are receiving palliative and end of life care is an essential part of the nurse's role. As a student nurse it is tempting to focus on addressing the physical symptoms people have as these tend to be tangible: something we can see, understand and manage. An example of this could be nausea and vomiting; we can review the person's medicine chart and administer the prescribed antiemetic, usually with good effect. Holistic care in palliative and end of life care, however, is much more than physical symptom management. It is the recognition that a person is not just a body, but is a 'whole' person with a mind, body and spirit that are interconnected in a way that affects the individual's sense of well-being and 'hope'. The key principles of palliative and end of life care emphasise the need for psychological, emotional and spiritual support (National Institute for Clinical Excellence (NICE) 2004) in addition to effective physical symptom management. While these principles relate to people living with cancer, this support should be available to all people who are living with a life-threatening condition. This emphasis on holistic care requires nurses to be self-aware and to work with people, their carers and families to ensure the delivery of person-centred care.

Defining holistic care

Holistic nursing care embraces the mind, body and spirit of the patient, in a culture that supports a therapeutic nurse/patient relationship, resulting in wholeness, harmony and healing. Holistic care is patient led and patient focused in order to provide individualised care, thereby, caring for the patient as a whole person rather than in fragmented parts.
(McEvoy and Duffy 2008, p418)

The term holism comes from the Greek work *holos*, which means whole. Holistic care has been part of nursing practice for decades and can find its roots in humanist theories where patients were viewed as unique individuals continually interacting with their environment (Rogers 1970; Levine 1971). Today this means viewing the patient as a whole, recognising the interconnection between the physical, social, cultural and spiritual aspects and the impact that illness can have on these (McEvoy and Duffy 2008). In their concept analysis of holistic nursing practice, McEvoy and Duffy (2008) identified the following recurring characteristics of holism:

- mind – the emotional and social aspect of a person;
- body – the physical aspect of a person;
- spirit – the spiritual and cultural aspect of a person;
- whole – recognising the person as a whole and the interrelation between mind, body and spirit;
- harmony – working in partnership with the patient;
- healing – recognising what is important to the patient and addressing these aspects.

The following case study illustrates how these characteristics relate to holistic care.

Case study

Margaret was an 84-year-old woman who lived in a residential home; she had lived there for the past three years. She had a fall where she injured her leg. The District Nurse (DN) was asked to review and dress Margaret's wound. This is the DN's narrative from this meeting.

When I met Margaret for the first time the first thing she said to me was 'I'm sorry that I'm not dressed' (mind and spirit). She went on to explain that she felt awkward in her nightgown and dressing gown (spirit). I apologised for my early visit and asked if she was happy for me to carry on, which she was (harmony and healing). My first thought was: 'How can I make her feel more at ease?' I got a blanket from her bed and placed it over her knees (mind and spirit, harmony and healing). Margaret smiled at this gesture (harmony). I then asked Margaret if there was a better time for me to visit so she would be dressed when I visited (mind, body and spirit and harmony). I went on to explain the reason for my visit, to review and dress her wound (body, healing and harmony).

As I prepared my equipment Margaret and I began to chat. I explained that as this was my first visit I would need to ask some questions and undertake an assessment (harmony). I began to clean the wound on Margaret's leg (body and healing), explaining as I went along what I was observing for (healing and harmony). Gradually Margaret began to relax and we talked about other things (harmony). It was clear Margaret was keen to talk: she was worried about her condition, she was feeling more tired and her recent fall had shaken her (mind, body and spirit). I asked Margaret what she thought this might mean. She replied: 'I know I'm not going to live forever, but I worry this change means things are getting worse, I don't know how to talk to Grace about it' (spirit and whole). Grace, I found out, was her long-term partner. Grace still lived in the house they shared and had been Margaret's carer until her own health prevented her caring for Margaret (mind, spirit and harmony).

As I bandaged Margaret's leg (body), I asked her if she would like to talk to Grace about the future and what that might mean. I said I would be happy to be with her when she did (mind, body and spirit, healing and harmony). Margaret's face relaxed at this suggestion (mind and spirit); the thought of having someone there to help answer questions was something she obviously found comforting.

There can be an assumption that holistic care and 'knowing' your patients is more beneficial to them and the care you deliver. This may not always be the case. Not everyone will wish to discuss their social, cultural and spiritual lives. They may feel it is not necessary to their care; indeed, they may feel it is intrusive. It is important therefore that you know the people you are nursing and how much they are prepared to share with you. You can see from the case study above that the nurse allowed Margaret to lead the conversation. When discussing more personal aspects with patients it is important that you consider why you are seeking this information and what, if any, impact this has on the care you deliver (Smart 2005).

Activity 2.1   *Reflection*

Using a reflection from your clinical practice that was based on a patient interaction, integrate the characteristics of holism (mind, body, spirit, whole, harmony and healing) to your reflection.

Brief answers to all activities are given at the end of the chapter, unless otherwise indicated. This activity is based on your own observations, so there is no outline answer given.

You can see from Activity 2.1 that the relationship between the technical care provided and how this care is carried out is central to holistic care. Once you recognise the importance of both these aspects your care will include both the science and art of nursing.

You will be aware of the importance of assessment in relation to providing person-centred care. It is part of the nursing process and forms the basis for your nursing interventions. This is no different in palliative and end of life care. The next part of this chapter focuses on assessment and how you can assess patients' holistic needs to support them towards a 'good' death.

Assessing for holistic care

The purpose of assessing people for their palliative and end of life care needs is to make sure that the care you provide helps them to maintain quality of life. Assessment tools provide you with a person-centred framework that you can use to guide your assessment. However, it is how you use them that will ensure the most effective assessment. Effective use of assessment tools requires you to have developed a positive therapeutic relationship and includes the use of effective communication skills, such as asking open questions, paraphrasing and using active listening skills (see Chapter 3 for further information on communication skills in palliative and end of life care).

When to assess

This is not always an easy decision to make. To support decision making the Gold Standards Framework (GSF) has introduced guidance to support health care professionals about when to introduce palliative and end of life care for people who have advanced disease (GSF 2006). There are three triggers that can be used to identify these people:

1. The surprise question: 'Would you be surprised if this person were to die in the next 6–12 months?' If the answer to this question is no, then begin to assess for palliative and end of life care.
2. Choice/need: the person with advanced disease makes a *choice* for comfort care only, not 'curative' treatment, or is in special *need* of supportive/palliative care.
3. Clinical indicators: specific indicators of advanced disease are present, e.g., in chronic obstructive pulmonary disease (COPD), more than three admissions to hospital in the last 12 months due to exacerbation of the patient's COPD and fulfils the criteria for long-term oxygen therapy.

To support the use of the above triggers it is useful for you to have an understanding of the different disease trajectories.

Research summary

Differing disease trajectories can make planning for palliative and end of life care challenging. Research by Lunney et al. (2002) examined disease trajectories at end of life to determine if a person's functional decline differed depending on their type of illness. The four causes of death included were: sudden death, death from cancer, death from organ failure and frailty and cognitive decline. The results of their study concluded that functional decline varied at end of life depending on the illness. Their results showed that one of the most unpredictable trajectories was for organ failure. The disease trajectory in these cases is identified by episodes of exacerbation followed by periods of stabilisation with some functional decline in health. This makes giving a prognosis difficult. This is highlighted by the fact that most people with heart failure die when doctors have expected them to live for more than six months (Murray and Sheikh 2008). This can mean that patients with organ failure are not always referred appropriately to palliative care services.

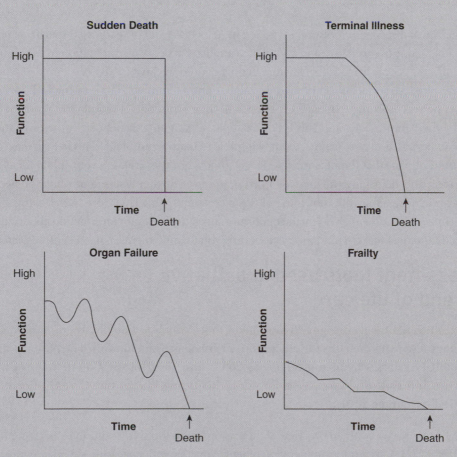

Figure 2.1: Trajectories of dying (Lunney et al. 2002).

Understanding disease trajectories in palliative and end of life care will help you to plan for and implement palliative and end of life care appropriately. Once a person has been identified as being suitable for palliative and end of life care it is important to undertake a holistic assessment of that person's needs.

Why holistic assessment is important

This activity will prompt you to consider the assessment tools you have used in your clinical practice.

Activity 2.2   *Reflection*

Reflect back on your clinical experience and answer the following points:

* List the assessment tools you have used in your clinical experience.
* Review this list and identify the assessment tools that assess specific care needs, e.g. pain assessment, wound assessment.
* Identify what assessment tools you have used that assess a person's holistic needs.

An outline answer is given at the end of the chapter.

The majority of assessment tools you identified in Activity 2.2 will have assessed specific care needs. For patients requiring palliative and end of life care these types of assessment often miss important aspects of care. People living with a life-threatening condition can experience a range of symptoms, including physical, social and spiritual ones (Maher and Hemming 2005). Living with these symptoms can be very isolating: patients' experience of their symptoms is unique to them and is influenced by their mind, body and spirit. For example, a patient with financial worries (mind) may begin to experience anxiety (spirit) about being able to pay the mortgage. This in turn may increase the amount of pain that the person experiences (body). In this situation your initial focus may be on assessing and managing the increase in pain; however further assessment would be needed to identify and address fully the root cause of this increase in pain. Therefore undertaking a holistic person-centred assessment gives you the opportunity to gather relevant information about a patient's care needs and personal circumstances, supporting you to implement a person-centred plan of care.

Assessment tools used in palliative and end of life care

There are two nationally recognised assessment tools, which will be discussed here. It is recognised that these form the basis for other more regional assessment tools. The national tools are the PEPSICOLA assessment tool (Thomas 2003) and the Holistic Common Assessment of Supportive and Palliative Care Needs for Adults Requiring End of Life Care (National End of Life Care Programme 2010).

Table 2.1 provides you with an overview of these assessment tools. In addition to assessing the 'personal', PEPSICOLA takes into consideration other factors that influence care, e.g. what happens in an emergency. Including these areas as part of your assessment can help communication, coordination and continuity of care (Thomas 2003). Before gathering any information it is important to gain consent for the assessment to take place. In preparation for the assessment you might want to find out what previous assessments have been done and identify any key points from these. It is important to find out if the person is able to participate in the assessment, and if not how that person's wishes are going to inform the assessment and to find out if the patient would like a family member present. Relevant background information, including the following, should also be used in the assessment:

- demographic information;
- carer and dependent information;
- preferred language for communication (written and verbal);
- previous medical history;
- allergies;
- medication;
- lifestyle (smoking, diet, etc.);
- professionals involved in care.

Including this information in your initial assessment ensures that for future assessments you have access to this information. This reduces the number of questions that need to be asked and supports continuity of care.

PEPSICOLA	**Consider:**	**Holistic Common Assessment**	**Consider:**
Physical	- Assessment of symptoms - Overall management plan - Medication, both regular and PRN - Stopping non-essential treatment/medication - Treatment/medication side-effects	Physical well-being; the aim is to identify all potential need; a review of all aspects of physical health is required	Identify the priority need/s: - Ask for a description of the problem: Was there a specific cause? How long has it lasted? Is it there all the time? Is it changing? What makes it better? - Find out the effect of this on the person and his/her level of activity - Identify what has been tried to manage this, e.g. medication, self care - Discuss with the patient if current management is working - Find out any further needs - Explore any fears/anxieties

(Continued)

(Continued)

PEPSICOLA	Consider:	Holistic Common Assessment	Consider:
Emotional	• What does the patient know about his/her illness? • What is the patient's emotional reaction to the diagnosis? • How are family and friends coping? • Are there signs of clinical depression? • Does the patient have any dependents? • What signifies a deterioration? What is to be expected?	Psychological well-being: the recognition of psychological needs, not specialist assessment	The following prompts should be used: • Ask for a description of the problem • Find out the history of the problem: is this usual? • What impact is this having on the person? • What impact is this having on others? • What strategies has the patient used? • Are these helping? • Does anything else need to be done?
Personal	• Cultural background, language, sexuality, spiritual and religious needs	Spiritual well-being: it is important to lead in to this assessment. If you do not feel comfortable undertaking this assessment, then ask another member of the HCT	Prior to assessing this aspect of a patient's care you should already know the patient's cultural background. Aspects to include: • An initial discussions to find out the patient's existing faith/belief – this may not be religious or conventional • Identify the patient's worries/challenges. Has the diagnosis impacted on the patient's faith? • Identify the patient's needs in relation to spiritual well-being • Are there any restrictions related to the patient's spirituality or diet? • Does the patient have any life goals that he/she would like to achieve?

PEPSICOLA	Consider:	Holistic Common Assessment	Consider:
Social	• Social care assessment • Carer assessment • What aids are required? • What is the person's preferred place of care?	Social and occupational well-being; home and community, work and finance, family and close relations and social and recreational	In relation to the four subdomains discuss the following: • The patient's general situation • Are there any restrictions/limitations? • What support is the person receiving? Is this sufficient? • Are there any additional needs?
Information and communication	• From the person and family to the health care team (HCT) and vice versa • Communication between members of the HCT • Patient-held records • Communication – is the person aware of the plans? Does he/she understand them? • Is communication appropriate?		
Control and autonomy	Assess: • Mental capacity • Treatment options • Preferred priorities of care • Advance care planning • Is there conflict between the wishes of the patient and those of the carer?		
Out of hours	• Communication – between HCT and out of hours – does the person know whom to contact? • Carer support • Medication support • Medication		

(Continued)

(Continued)

PEPSICOLA	Consider:	Holistic Common Assessment	Consider:
Late	End of life/terminal care (last two days): • Is the person comfortable with good symptom control? • Are the person and family aware of the situation? • Has all non-essential medication been stopped?		
Aftercare	• Planning for bereavement • Provide information to the family • Inform other members of the HCT of the death		

Table 2.1: Areas to consider when undertaking a holistic assessment of a person's palliative and end of life care needs when using either PEPSICOLA (Thomas 2003) or the Holistic Common Assessment (National End of Life Care Programme 2010)

Case study

Fred is 69 years old; he has hypertension (diagnosed 15 years ago). Fred has had four myocardial infarctions in the past two years and now has heart failure. Fred has been married to Mavis for 49 years; they are very close and, until Fred's health started to deteriorate, did everything together. Fred and Mavis are becoming socially isolated, Fred as a result of his illness and Mavis because she does not like to leave Fred. Their two sons live some distance away and visit twice a year. Neither Fred nor Mavis wants to bother them. They would like to talk to them about their situation but don't know what to say.

Fred and Mavis live in a rented first-floor flat; neither of them drives. Mavis relies on the local shop for food, though her neighbour takes her shopping to the supermarket once a fortnight. Fred worked as a self-employed painter and decorator and only receives his state pension. Mavis looked after the house and brought up their sons. Fred feels the cold easily; recently they have had to have the heating on more frequently. They are both concerned about the cost of the heating.

Fred has smoked since he was 14 and has never tried to stop. He is overweight. This impacts on his mobility; he is not able to go up and down stairs and Mavis has to help him with his personal hygiene and dressing. Fred is increasingly breathless and has begun to complain of generalised musculoskeletal pain. His breathlessness worsened after an admission to hospital with a chest infection which has left him feeling fatigued. This was his second hospital admission in four months. Fred was provided with equipment following his admission: a urinal, commode and perching stool. Mavis, despite wanting to care for Fred herself, is finding it increasingly difficult getting Fred up and out of bed. Both Fred and Mavis are concerned about his deteriorating health, and have questions to ask. Fred would like to know how long he has left and is worried that caring for him is too much for Mavis. Mavis's main worry is about what to do in an emergency.

Fred takes the following medication:

- *Bumetanide 2mg mané*
- *Enalapril 5mg*
- *Bisoprolol 5mg*
- *Lactulose 15mg TID*

Fred's care is coordinated by his community matron (Debbie) who liaises with his GP. Both Fred's GP and Debbie are concerned about his deteriorating condition and have asked each other the 'surprise question': 'Would you be surprised if Fred were to die in the next 6–12 months?' They both answered no. In the past Fred and Mavis have refused offers of support at home. This is Debbie's first visit to Fred and Mavis since the GP spoke to them about Fred's future care. Debbie would like to use this visit to assess Fred and Mavis's needs so that she can begin to plan their care.

Activity 2.3   *Critical thinking*

Use the PEPSICOLA and Holistic Common Assessment frameworks to assess Fred and Mavis's needs in relation to palliative and end of life care.

An outline answer is given at the end of this chapter.

Activity 2.3 has allowed you to carry out a holistic assessment; you may not have felt confident in assessing all aspects of Fred's care. If you did not, you must recognise this and discuss this with other members of the clinical team. We will use this assessment to identify one area of Fred's care that requires ongoing care planning and management.

Symptom management in palliative and end of life care

To allow you to explore and understand the holistic management of symptoms in palliative and end of life care we will focus on Fred's dyspnoea. Dyspnoea is a recognised and well-reported symptom of heart failure. Albert et al. (2010) reported that in heart failure dyspnoea was one of the top five reported symptoms. Dyspnoea can be a real and distressing symptom for patients and their carer/family. Patients often describe their dyspnoea like 'breathing through a straw'. If you have tried to breathe through a straw and carry out any activity, you will understand how restrictive this must be. Recent discussions in palliative care have suggested that the concept of 'total dyspnoea' (Abernethy and Wheeler 2008) be recognised, much like the concept of 'total pain' (Saunders et al. 1995). This recognises that dyspnoea is unique to individuals and is influenced by their physical, emotional, social and spiritual well-being. Using the nursing process will provide you with a clear framework to use when implementing a plan of care to manage Fred's dyspnoea.

Using the nursing process for effective symptom management in palliative and end of life care

The nursing process is an essential theme in the *Standards for Pre-registration Nursing Education* (Nursing and Midwifery Council 2010). Initially this process incorporated four steps: assess, plan, implement and evaluate; over time this has been adapted and refined. A further two steps have been added (Barrett et al. 2009). The steps in the nursing process are now:

- Assess
- Systematic nursing diagnosis
- Plan
- Implement
- Recheck
- Evaluate.

This can be remembered by the acronym ASPIRE. When using the nursing process it is important to remember that all steps are interrelated. You cannot put an effective plan in place unless you have carried out a holistic assessment and a systematic nursing diagnosis has been made. In turn your plan cannot be rechecked and evaluated if you have not implemented one. You have already undertaken an assessment of Fred and his dyspnoea has been identified as a priority. You can now plan and implement care to manage this; the first step would be to consider some of the causes of Fred's dyspnoea. This may be due to changes in his skeletal and respiratory muscles (physical) resulting in increased effort, and this would tie in with his generalised musculoskeletal pain. However Fred's dyspnoea could be exacerbated by his concerns about his future (spiritual) and the impact his deteriorating health is having on Mavis (emotional). Table 2.2 details the possible care and management you might implement to address Fred's dyspnoea.

Nursing process	Application to Fred's increased dyspnoea
Assess	Fred's needs have been assessed using the PEPSICOLA framework: • Increasing dyspnoea following recent chest infection • Increased dyspnoea could be due to generalised musculoskeletal pain • Take into consideration emotional, social and spiritual factors that could increase Fred's dyspnoea, e.g. his concern about Mavis and her ability to manage caring for him

Nursing process	Application to Fred's increased dyspnoea
Systematic nursing diagnosis	To reduce the level of dyspnoea experienced by Fred to a level that he finds manageable and that maintains his sense of well-being
Plan	1. Assess and treat reversible causes – undertake a complete pain assessment 2. Review medication and confirm that Fred is taking this correctly, optimising efficacy 3. Discuss with Fred his financial situation 4. Manage Fred and Mavis's expectations
Implement	1. Prescribe regular simple analgesia (paracetamol QID). Asking Fred to complete a pain diary will assist you in rechecking and evaluating the care implemented 2. Review diuretic. This could be taken BD to allow for more effective management of any oedema 3. Ensure that relevant benefits are being claimed; with Fred's consent, refer to social services for review. To address Fred's anxiety about Mavis, ensure that a carer assessment is completed 4. Provide education about self-help methods: pacing activity to minimise dyspnoea; a fan can have a calming effect. It may also be appropriate to prescribe short-acting opioids. As Fred is not currently taking any opiate medication, start with a low dose of 2.5 mg oral morphine sulphate PRN for dyspnoea. Discuss with Fred his symptoms and what these signify in relation to his health. It would be appropriate to discuss Fred's future care needs (advance care planning), especially in relation to further deterioration. Refer on to physiotherapist or occupational therapist for further coping strategies and equipment Asking Fred to keep a note of when he experiences dyspnoea and what factors lessen/exacerbate it will help you to recheck and evaluate the care implemented
Recheck	In the initial stages a recheck visit is planned for every three days to monitor the effectiveness of the care implemented. A formal evaluation will take place at the end of two weeks
Evaluate	The care implemented will be evaluated in relation to effective management of Fred's dyspnoea. Due to Fred's condition it is not likely that his dyspnoea will be completely resolved; however the aim would be for it to be manageable for both Fred and Mavis. Evaluation also allows for a critical analysis of the care-planning process: Was the pain assessment tool used appropriate? Was a holistic approach taken? Was the stated goal realistic? Were the interventions planned suitable for Fred and his needs?

Table 2.2: The nursing process (Barrett et al. 2009) applied to Fred's dyspnoea

As you will have seen from Table 2.2, using a holistic assessment framework allowed you to implement, recheck and evaluate a plan of care to address Fred's dyspnoea. The same process can now be used to implement a plan of care for other patients.

Activity 2.4   *Decision making*

Read again the case study of Johnny in Chapter 1.

You are spending the day with the Macmillan Clinical Nurse Specialist (David) who is coordinating Johnny's care. This is David's third visit to see Johnny and Sandra; he has already completed a holistic assessment and has implemented a plan of care to address Johnny's care needs. However Johnny is now experiencing fatigue and David asks you to use the nursing process to compile a holistic plan of care to address this care need.

The article by Hawthorn (2010) listed in the further reading section in this chapter will provide you with useful information to assist you in planning and implementing care to manage Johnny's fatigue.

An outline answer is given at the end of this chapter.

Activities 2.3 and 2.4 provided you with the opportunity to assess and plan holistic care for a patient receiving palliative and end of life care. Within this there is recognition of the importance of the body, mind and spirit and how they contribute to a patient's overall sense of health and well-being. This is especially true for people facing their own mortality, when maintaining a sense of hope is crucial (see Chapter 4 for further information relating to Kübler Ross and her work on dying):

> *You matter to us because **you are you**, and you matter to the last moment of your life. We will do all we can not only to help you die peacefully, but also to live until you die.*
> (Dame Cicely Saunders; emphasis added)

This quote emphasises the uniqueness of the person and the need to care for the whole person, not just the disease and symptoms.

Spirituality as part of holistic care

Nursing has always incorporated art and science; it is the utilisation of both these aspects in your practice that allows you to *nurse*. The art of nursing recognises the human nature of nursing, of 'being with' the patients you are nursing. Focusing on the *whole* person, getting involved and developing a therapeutic relationship all contribute to the patient feeling valued and humanised (Clarke 2013). While the art of nursing informs *how* you practise, the science of nursing informs *why* you practise by recognising the role that knowledge and skill acquisition have in supporting the care provided.

However, there is a tendency to address spirituality as a need in the way you would assess a patient's mobility (Clarke 2013). You might ask, 'What religion are you?' followed up by, 'Would you like the chaplain to visit you?' If this approach is used and a need identified, 'Yes, I would like the chaplain to visit', this aspect of the person's care is then handed over to the chaplain, the need having been met. This is a limited and rather narrow approach, especially in the context of holistic care and nursing the mind, body and spirit. Acknowledging the uniqueness of individuals, recognising the importance of caring for the whole person, mind, body and spirit, will support you to deliver compassionate care. In palliative and end of life care, assessment frameworks such as PEPSICOLA and the Common Holistic Assessment framework ensure that spiritual assessment is an integral part of any assessment.

Defining spirituality

Spirituality, by its very nature, is nebulous and difficult to define. Due to the personal nature of spirituality there are arguments for and against trying to define it (Ellis and Narayanasamy 2009). However, providing a definition does give a starting point for exploring spirituality as part of holistic palliative and end of life care. Ross (1996) defines spirituality as:

> *The need to find meaning, purpose and fulfillment in life, suffering and death. The need for hope and the will to live, the need for belief and faith in self, others and a power beyond self or God as defined by the individual.*

Activity 2.5   *Reflection*

Using the definition above as a starting point, write down what spirituality means to you and how this contributes to your body, mind and spirit.

As this activity is based on your own observations, there is no outline answer at the end of this chapter.

Your response to Activity 2.5 will be unique and personal to you; this is the same for your patients. You may also have identified that spirituality is more than religion, that it emphasises the essence, soul and meaning in your life. For some, though, religion does have a strong influence on their spirituality and life. Religion offers people a framework, allowing them to express their spirituality and, for some people, may provide answers to important questions about life and death (Govier 2000). Yet within religious groups there will be different interpretations. You may be caring for patients who, when asked, state they are Christian; however, what this means to them, their life and sense of self will be different for each of them. One may state that being Christian is about adhering to the ten commandments, for another it may be regular attendance at church and the sense of community this brings, yet for another it may be that prayer is an important aspect of Christianity. This will be the same for other religious faiths, e.g. Islam. One patient may say that wearing a *khimaar* is an important part of her faith, another that observing *salat* provides his life with a sense of meaning and purpose. Recognising the individual nature of spirituality and incorporating this into your nursing practice allows you to adjust the care you provide to reflect individual patient beliefs, e.g. providing them with a place to pray, supporting them to attend church.

To support the delivery of spiritual care nurses need to be confident, yet it is known that nurses have a lack of confidence in this aspect of care (McSherry and Jamieson 2011). Increasing your understanding about spirituality will support you to develop your own knowledge and understanding. One model you could use to develop your knowledge and understanding of spiritual care could be the ASSET model (Actioning Spirituality and Spiritual care Education and Training in nursing) (Ellis and Narayanasamy 2009) (Figure 2.2).

Self-awareness

- What are my personal beliefs, values, prejudices, assumptions and feelings?
- How may these influence the way in which I nurse?

↓

Spirituality

- What does holistic care mean to me?
- What other beliefs are there?
- What do I know about different belief systems, including religious, humanist and secularist?

↓

Spiritual nursing (reflection on patient care – some trigger questions)

- Have I considered what things are important in this patient's life?
- Am I open to verbal and non-verbal cues?
- How does the patient relate to others? Who are the important people in the patient's life and how does she/he respond to them?
- Is the patient displaying possible signs of spiritual distress?
- Is the patient displaying any evidence of religious affiliation (symbols, texts, etc.)?
- Am I facilitating a trusting, open nurse–patient relationship?
- Am I providing the patient with privacy as well as the opportunity to talk and express feelings?
- Am I able to provide holistic care or is a multidisciplinary approach required (e.g. chaplain, social worker)?
- Have I evaluated any spiritual intervention?

Figure 2.2: An adapted version of the ASSET model (Narayanasamy 2006; cited in Ellis and Narayanasamy 2009).

Activity 2.6   *Reflection*

Using your answer from Activity 2.5 and the ASSET model, reflect on a recent patient you have nursed and answer the questions posed by the ASSET model.

As this activity is based on your own observations, there is no outline answer at the end of this chapter.

Activity 2.6 will have allowed you to explore your knowledge and attitude in relation to incorporating spiritual care into your nursing practice. It will have encouraged you to reflect on the knowledge and skills required, e.g. the use of non-verbal communication such as touch. It may also have identified some of the barriers that may be present.

Barriers to talking about spirituality

Much has been written about the barriers present when talking about spirituality (McSherry 2006). Barriers can be patient-focused, e.g. an inability to communicate due to the patient's illness. This may be due to dysphasia or loss of cognitive function. This can result in spiritual needs not being acknowledged and met. Your plan should be to find alternative ways to communicate, perhaps in writing or using pictures. In some cases you may have to discuss with other family members what is important to the patient. Barriers can be nurse-focused, e.g. a lack of knowledge about spirituality might lead to a lack of confidence. Being clear about what you, and what the patient, mean when talking about spirituality can improve confidence. In addition if you are both clear at the start it is more likely that you will provide spiritually appropriate care for that patient. You might feel it is too sensitive to discuss; you may be worried that once the conversation starts you will not be able to answer the questions asked. Being self-aware and knowing when to stop and whom to contact if questions become awkward are important parts of ensuring trust between you and the patient. This can be especially true in palliative and end of life care where patients ask questions such as 'Why me?', 'Am I being punished for something I have done?' or 'If there is a God, then why is this happening?'

The clinical environment can also produce barriers, e.g. a lack of privacy or time. Providing quiet areas where patients can discuss personal aspects of their care ensures that conversations about spirituality can take place. The perception can be that discussing spirituality takes up a lot of time. This is not necessarily the case: it can take place while other nursing care is being done, e.g. while assisting a person to have a bath, with your use of touch providing spiritual comfort.

The use of touch to promote spiritual care

Much nursing care is described as 'hands on' and this term has endured throughout the history of nursing (Engebretson 2002). You are 'hands on' when washing somebody, 'hands on' when dressing a wound and 'hands on' when comforting someone late at night. It is this physical aspect of nursing that presents the ideal opportunity for spiritual care to become integral to your nursing care (Clarke 2013). This approach moves away from spiritual care being a 'need' to 'assess' to spiritual care being the 'essence' of the nursing care you provide. This does not mean that assessing and addressing spirituality is not important; both approaches can be used to allow you to encompass spiritual care in your nursing practice. Touch is an integral part of this care: with touch you are reaching out to someone, perhaps more than you would with words or eye contact. By reaching out you are not only making a physical connection with the person, you are also implying that you are *with them* (Clarke 2013).

The more support a patient requires in carrying out daily activities, the more 'touch' will occur. Some of the most common nursing interventions require what is termed 'intimate care': care of the parts of our bodies that we usually care for ourselves – breasts, genitals, buttocks. Touching these parts of a patient's body may cause anxiety for you and for the patient. Research by O'Lynn and Krautscheid (2011) focused on exploring how you should touch patients when carrying out intimate care. Their research identified four recurring themes: 'communicate with me', 'give me choices', 'ask me about gender' and 'touch me professionally, not too fast and not too slow'. Table 2.3 summarises these themes and relates them to spiritual care.

Theme	Summary of theme	Relevance to spiritual care
'Communicate with me'	<ul><li>Talk to the patient before touching him/her</li><li>Find out what the patient would like to be called</li><li>Ask for the patient's permission to carry out the activity</li><li>Explain what is going to happen</li><li>Make eye contact, if appropriate, and talk to the patient</li><li>Develop a rapport with the patient</li><li>The use of humour is appropriate</li></ul>	<ul><li>Fosters trust</li><li>Recognises individuality, empowers patients and shows them you respect their contribution</li><li>Respects their wishes, demonstrates care and makes them feel central to your care</li><li>Makes them feel cared for because you are focusing your attention on them</li><li>Demonstrates you are interested in them and value their contribution, displays empathy</li></ul>
'Give me choices'	<ul><li>Ask what the patient wants; do not assume</li><li>Involve the patient in the decision making</li><li>Explore alternatives</li></ul>	<ul><li>Recognises patients' value; increases their sense of self-esteem</li><li>Demonstrates respect for them and their choices</li></ul>
'Ask me about gender'	<ul><li>Ask patients if they mind if the nurse is male/female</li><li>Be professional and competent</li><li>Consider the use of chaperones</li></ul>	<ul><li>Respects patients' choices and decisions; reinforces that they have a contribution to make</li><li>Shows sensitivity to their feelings</li></ul>
'Touch me professionally, not too fast and not too slow'	<ul><li>Make eye contact</li><li>Ensure privacy, keep doors closed</li><li>Minimal exposure</li><li>Taking your time to touch but not too much time</li><li>Asking for feedback</li></ul>	<ul><li>Attention is demonstrated: this may encourage patients to talk about other concerns they may have</li><li>Displays respect and empathy</li><li>Provides security, may help the person to relax</li><li>Is sensitive to their feelings</li></ul>

Table 2.3: Using touch to integrate spiritual care into everyday nursing practice (using themes from O'Lynn and Krautscheid 2011)

Activity 2.7   *Reflection*

Using the themes in Table 2.3 to structure your reflection, reflect on a situation where you have been providing intimate care for a patient.

As this activity is based on your own observations, there is no outline answer at the end of this chapter.

Activity 2.7 will have allowed you to see how touch can promote spiritual care as part of your nursing practice; you may have identified areas for further development. This approach can foster feelings of self-worth and security which can provide a sense of reassurance, a sense of belonging and connection with the world around.

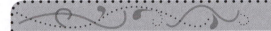

Chapter summary

This chapter has provided you with an overview of holistic care in palliative and end of life care. The term holistic care has been explored and the need for nursing to nurse the mind, body and spirit has been related to a case scenario. There has been a focus on the importance of holistic assessment to ensure that the needs of the person, and his or her carer/family, at end of life are identified and met. The nursing process has been used to support the delivery of holistic care and effective symptom management. Specific strategies have been identified and discussed to support this process, e.g. PEPSICOLA and the nursing process. The importance of recognising spirituality and spiritual care and how to integrate this into your everyday nursing practice have been explored.

Activities: brief outline answers

Activity 2.2: Reflection

You might have used the following assessment tools: observation chart (specific: S), activities of daily living assessment (holistic: H), falls risk assessment (S), Waterlow risk assessment (S), MUST assessment (S), pain assessment (S), Glasgow Coma Scale (S) and Depression Rating Scale (S).

Activity 2.3: critical thinking

PEPSICOLA	Holistic Common Assessment	Application to Fred and Mavis
Physical	Physical well-being	Assessment of Fred's physical symptoms, including pain and breathlessness. Due to Fred's pain a pain assessment should be carried out. An assessment of Fred's breathlessness would need to be carried out using the Medical Research Council (MRC) dyspnoea scale (MRC 2007)

(Continued)

(Continued)

PEPSICOLA	Holistic Common Assessment	Application to Fred and Mavis
		Review of Fred's medication Discuss what steps Fred and Mavis have taken to manage Fred's pain and breathlessness and if these work Ask Fred and Mavis if they feel further support is required, e.g., hospital bed, carer support
Emotional	Psychological well-being	Fred and Mavis are aware that Fred's condition is deteriorating. They are concerned about what this means; both seem anxious. Fred would like to know how much time he has left and Mavis is concerned about what to do in an emergency. Fred worries that the physical aspect of caring for him is too much for Mavis. Discussions with Fred and Mavis may focus on what to do in an emergency; at this time preferred priorities of care could be discussed, and what support is needed. You could consider a pendant alarm for Fred in case of falls
Personal	Spiritual well-being	Fred does not mention any particular religious belief. It is evident that Fred and Mavis have a close relationship. Discussing this with them would be appropriate, e.g. how do they maintain their closeness with each other? Are there things that Fred finds particularly comforting, e.g. listening to music? As Fred's sons live away it might be that Fred would like to see them before his condition deteriorates further. Mavis feels her role is to care for Fred, but she is finding this increasingly difficult. Both Fred and Mavis may have feelings of guilt in relation to this; this could impact on their sense of 'self', who they are and what is important to them
Social	Social and occupational well-being	Due to Fred's financial situation, he is concerned about their heating bills. Ensure that they are claiming all available benefits. Has a DS1500 been completed? Refer to social services for a carer assessment. Find out from Fred his preferred place of care
Information and communication		Make sure that Fred has a copy of his notes; do other members of the health care team know where to find them? Are Fred and Mavis aware of what is happening and whom to contact?

PEPSICOLA	Holistic Common Assessment	Application to Fred and Mavis
Control and autonomy		Mavis is keen to care for Fred for as long as possible. It would be appropriate to find out if Fred would like to die at home and how Mavis feels about this
Out of hours		Both Fred and Mavis need to know whom to contact in an emergency. It will be important to ensure that out of hours staff know about Fred and what to do in case of a deterioration
Late		Aspects addressed in relation to social support and control and autonomy
Aftercare		It may be worth discussing if Fred has thought about funeral arrangements. Is there anything he would particularly like to have?

Activity 2.4: Decision making

Nursing process	Application to Johnny's fatigue
Assess	Johnny's needs have been assessed using the PEPSICOLA framework: • Johnny is reporting fatigue; this is a new symptom • Take into consideration the impact Johnny's fatigue could have on his emotional, social and spiritual needs, e.g. his wish to see the birth of his first grandchild and his love of bikes
Systematic nursing diagnosis	To reduce the level of fatigue experienced by Johnny to a level that he finds manageable and that maintains his sense of well-being
Plan	1. To assess and treat reversible causes 2. To assess and treat any clinical depression 3. To assess Johnny's sleep pattern. Ask him to keep a sleep diary that includes: How easy is it for you to fall asleep? Do you manage to stay asleep or do you wake during the night and are then unable to go back to sleep? Do you wake feeling refreshed or not? Are you sleepy during the day? 4. To discuss with Johnny and Sandra what additional support they may need to help Johnny to conserve his energy, especially in light of Johnny's determination to take care of himself 5. To discuss with Johnny the impact his fatigue is having on his emotional and spiritual well-being

(Continued)

(Continued)

Nursing process	Application to Johnny's fatigue
Implement	1. Undertake a health assessment. Take a full blood count and urea and electrolytes to exclude reversible causes such as anaemia 2. Using the depression screening questions ('During the past month have you often been bothered by feeling down, depressed or hopeless?' and 'During the last month have you often been bothered by having little interest or pleasure in doing things?') recommended by NICE (2009). Consider whether referral on for further assessment is required 3. Review Johnny's sleep pattern and identify causes of problems if appropriate. For example, if he is coughing at night then implement a plan of care to manage his nocturnal cough (simple linctus, small-dose oral short-acting opioid) 4. Discuss the need to conserve energy. Carrying out tasks in stages and pacing activity may help. Providing aids that maximise function and minimise effort are an important aspect of managing fatigue; Johnny might be reluctant to consider these. Discussing this with Johnny and explaining the benefits in relation to conserving energy for use on the 'value added' things he likes to do might encourage him to think about this. Equipment that is available includes perching stool, commode and leg raisers 5. Discuss the importance of his bond with his fellow Hell's Angels and what this means to him and Sandra. Effective planning to allow Johnny to carry on going out with his fellow Angels, such as assessing for walking aids, providing information to his friends and contact numbers to phone if there is an emergency, will all contribute to Johnny's overall sense of well-being and hope
Recheck	In the initial stages a recheck visit is planned for every three days to monitor the effectiveness of the care implemented. A formal evaluation will take place at the end of two weeks
Evaluate	The care implemented will be evaluated in relation to effective management of Johnny's fatigue. Due to Johnny's condition it is not likely that his fatigue will be completely resolved; however the aim would be for it to be manageable. Evaluation also allows for a critical analysis of the care-planning process: Was a holistic approach taken? Was the stated goal realistic? Were the interventions planned suitable to Johnny and his needs?

Further reading

Clarke, J. (2013) *Spiritual Care in Everyday Nursing Practice: A New Approach.* Basingstoke: Palgrave Macmillan.

This book emphasises the need for spiritual care to be integral to holistic nursing care.

Middleton-Green, L. (2008) Managing total pain at the end of life: a case study analysis. *Nursing Standard,* 23 (6): 41–46.

This case analysis explores the individual total pain experience and how this was managed in a hospice setting.

Hawthorn, M. (2010) Fatigue in patients with advanced cancer. *International Journal of Palliative Nursing,* 16 (11): 536–541.

This article focuses on the assessment and management of cancer-related fatigue.

Nicol, J. (2011) *Nursing Adults with Long Term Conditions.* Exeter: Learning Matters.

This book has further information relating to the therapeutic relationship and emotional intelligence and symptom management.

Useful websites

http://www.e-lfh.org.uk/projects/end-of-life-care

This is the website for the End of Life Care strategy e-learning. Resources include advance care planning, assessment and symptom management.

www.nice.org.uk/mpc/index.jsp

This website, which combines the National Prescribing Centre and NICE, provides information to support the safe delivery of medicines.

www.npc.nhs.uk

This is the National Prescribing Centre archive website; while it is not being updated it does contain useful resources relating to patients and their medicines.

Chapter 3
Communication in palliative and end of life care

Jean Fisher

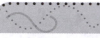

NMC Standards for Pre-registration Nursing Education

This chapter will address the following competencies:

Domain 2: Communication and interpersonal skills

2. All nurses must use a range of communication skills and technologies to support person-centred care and enhance quality and safety. They must ensure people receive all the information they need in a language and manner that allows them to make informed choices and share decision making. They must recognise when language interpretation or other communication support is needed and know how to obtain it.

Domain 4: Leadership, management and team working

6. All nurses must work independently as well as in teams. They must be able to take the lead in coordinating, delegating and supervising care safely, managing risk and remaining accountable for care given.

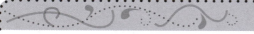

NMC Essential Skills Clusters

This chapter will address the following ESCs:

Cluster: Care, compassion and communication

5. People can trust the newly registered graduate nurse to engage with them in a warm, sensitive and compassionate manner.

By the first progression point

3. Interacts with the person in a manner that is interpreted as warm, sensitive, kind and compassionate, making appropriate use of touch.

By entry to the register

8. Listens to, watches for and responds to verbal and non-verbal cues.
9. Engages with people in the planning and provision of care that recognises personalised needs and provides practical and emotional support.

6. People can trust the newly registered graduate nurse to engage therapeutically and actively listen to their needs and concerns, responding using skills that are helpful, providing information that is clear, accurate, meaningful and free from jargon.

By the first progression point

1. Communicate effectively both orally and in writing so that the meaning is always clear.
4. Responds in a way that confirms what a person is communicating.

By entry to the register

8. Communicates effectively and sensitively in different settings using a range of methods and skills.
12. Uses the skills of active listening, questioning, paraphrasing and reflection to support a therapeutic intervention.

Cluster: Organisational aspects of care

14. People can trust the newly registered graduate nurse to be an autonomous and confident member of the multi-disciplinary or multi-agency team and to inspire confidence in others.

By the first progression point

1. Works within the Code (NMC 2008), and adheres to Guidance on professional conduct for nursing and midwifery students (NMC 2010).

By the second progression point

2. Values others' roles and responsibilities within the team and interacts appropriately.

Chapter aims

After reading this chapter you will be able to:

- appreciate the role emotional labour has in supporting key communication skills in palliative and end of life care;
- identify, describe and apply the key communication skills required in palliative and end of life care;
- recognise the role 'presence' can have in promoting effective communication in palliative and end of life care;
- understand potential communication barriers in palliative and end of life care and what strategies are available to reduce these.

Introduction

Rachel was a fit 37-year-old who developed a small lesion on her arm. She was encouraged by family members to 'get it checked out'. Having seen two GPs she was referred to a specialist dermatology service. She underwent biopsy and awaited results. She received a telephone call at work from the hospital consultant: 'I am sorry my dear, but as I feared this has turned out to be cancer, and I am afraid the horse has bolted.'

This phrase so stuck in her mind that she was able to repeat it to me verbatim four years later, just months before she died.

Activity 3.1   *Reflection*

Using the quote above and your own experience, think about and make brief notes on communication issues in palliative and end of life care situations that give you cause for concern. These may be issues you have encountered or witnessed, or things that you anticipate will be difficult if and when they arise. Consider why these particular scenarios concern you.

Brief answers to all activities are given at the end of the chapter, unless otherwise indicated. This activity is based on your own observations, so there is no outline answer given.

Although traditionally seen as being focused on cancer (Radbruch 2011), palliative and end of life care is a crucial component of long-term conditions management, e.g. in chronic obstructive pulmonary disease. Palliation may be needed for adults from the point of diagnosis of advanced disease, be that cancer or a non-malignant condition, or subsequent to a severe trauma or subarachnoid haemorrhage. Effective, person-centred communication in palliative and end of life care is relevant whether we care for pregnant or nursing mothers, a child with severe disabilities or a progressive illness, or elderly people with dementia.

Communication is at the heart of your nursing practice, and is the core of *The Code: Standards of Conduct, Performance and Ethics for Nurses and Midwives* (NMC 2008). The above quote and your reflection in Activity 3.1 highlight the complexity of the situations encountered in palliative and end of life care. Developing your knowledge and skills and exploring communication in palliative and end of life care will increase your confidence in this area and will support you to provide person-centred care. Effective communication enables you to assess pain and other symptoms accurately; to explore issues and concerns; to offer comfort and support to the dying person and his or her family and friends. Communication skills are pivotal to achieving true multidisciplinary practice in any arena of health care, and never more so than when you are caring for the very ill, the dying and the bereaved. It is recognised that often these situations and conversations can be emotional for both the patient and the nurse. Caring for a patient at the end of life calls for you to be prepared to undertake what is called emotional labour, which is the subject of the next section.

Emotional labour

The emotional labour of nursing was discussed by James (1989), as one of the necessary elements of care. Huynh et al. (2008) describe emotional labour as the internal regulation of emotions, which can be combined into the adoption of a 'work persona' in order to express or suppress emotions in patient encounters. It may be that, as a nurse, you experience conflict when caring for patients who have undergone radical treatment, yet still face death. Part of your role as a nurse is to invest in developing a therapeutic relationship with patients. Positivity and cheerfulness are usually valued by patients and families, as long as this is balanced by honesty. However, if the patient then becomes very ill, or dies, this carries a cost to you as a human being, as well as challenging your professional persona. It is crucial therefore that you develop some strategies that enable you to go on making that investment, whilst maintaining your own safety. Learning to strike that balance between the professional persona and the personal investment will involve reflection, clinical supervision and possibly other techniques such as mindfulness (Kabat Zinn 2011). Each of us needs to find our own way to manage compassion, caring, communication and coping, without resorting to distancing ourselves from the essential components of our everyday role as a nurse, including emotional labour.

Fundamental components of communication in palliative and end of life care

There are many constituents of communication; however the work of Mehrabian (1967) identified three fundamental ingredients within the 'communication cake'. This work identified that, for white Anglo-Saxons, body language is such a significant aspect that it represents more than half of the message conveyed. Body language consists of eye contact, body position and openness, e.g., whether your arms are crossed or relaxed by your side (Mehrabian 1967). In some cultures and countries body language may be very much more significant, e.g. the Italians utilise body language and hand gestures more than people in the UK. Cross-cultural significance of gestures can also differ: in Tibet the sticking out of the tongue is a greeting and is not considered to be rude. Tone represents over one-third of communication. Tone is the way you speak: is your tone harsh, encouraging, loud or soft? Finally, the words spoken account for only a small part of your communication. However the words you choose can mean more depending on if the communication is face to face and on the level of understanding a person has, e.g. when a patient has cognitive decline. Ensuring that your words are not ambiguous is also important: in palliative and end of life care, using terms such as 'passed over' and 'gone away' instead of 'died' may cause confusion at a time of emotional distress.

Mehrabian (1967) identified these proportions from research specifically in relation to feelings and attitudes, and he did not intend them to be seen as absolute or applying in all situations. Mehrabian (1967) and many others have noted the high level of importance attached to the congruence of messaging between the three aspects. If your words convey one message but your tone and body language convey another, then the message received may be mixed, or confused. For example, 'I am really sorry to hear about your mother's death' could be stated with clear eye contact and a warm tone. This would signal a genuine response. However the same words spoken in a dismissive tone and/or whilst looking at your watch demonstrate to the listener that actually you do not really care and/or that you are distracted by something else which you perceive as more important. Table 3.1 summarises aspects of body language and their potential significance in communication.

Element of body language	Potential message conveyed
Eye contact (EC)	Little EC may be seen as lack of interest
	Too much EC can be threatening and in some situations is better avoided. For example, some people with autistic spectrum disorder may find eye contact deeply distressing
Posture (P)	Closed P (crossed legs/arms etc.) may convey unfriendliness or rejection
	Open, relaxed P suggests warmth and friendliness
	Drooped head and shoulders may indicate depression or despair
	Muscular tension and stiffness can be signs of anxiety
Facial expression (FE)	FE conveys both emotion and attitudes. For people who cannot use facial expression, e.g. those with Parkinson's disease, opportunities to convey messages are compromised
Gestures (G)	G can be used to reinforce or emphasise certain points. Remember some people use gesticulation and shoulder shrugging much more. Furthermore, when caring for people from minority ethnic groups it is vital to consider how your non-verbal communication may be interpreted differently and the effect this might have on your relationship with that person

Table 3.1: Body language and its significance in communication

In a face-to-face conversation with a patient and/or family, when the words you use are perhaps less significant than you think, there is a high need for congruence in terms of your body language and tone. This is to ensure a clear and consistent meaning is received and understood by the person you are communicating with. However not all communication takes place face to face and you need to consider the implications of this for your practice.

Case study

Peter is an elderly married man with end-stage heart failure. He has been an inpatient on the ward where you are working for several weeks now and has steadily deteriorated. In fact Peter is dying. His very frail wife Amy visits daily and you have met her several times and had conversations both with her and with Peter and Amy together. She has spoken openly about her desire to be present when he finally dies. However, when Peter dies in his sleep Amy is at home. Your mentor asks you to phone Amy at home and give her the news of her husband's expected death.

Activity 3.2	*Communication*

Reflecting on the case study about Peter and Amy and considering the fundamental aspects of communication, answer the following:

- How would you feel about making this telephone call?
- What factors would you take into consideration?
- What fundamental aspects of communication would you need to pay attention to particularly in respect of how you communicate this news to Amy?
- How might the conversation be different if you were talking face to face with Amy?

An outline answer is given at the end of this chapter.

In Activity 3.2 you may have reflected on the difficulty of not being able to see Amy when breaking this news to her. We interpret and deduce much from people we are communicating with by *their* body language and tone too. This happens subconsciously and we are not necessarily aware of it. This can mean that we may 'misread the signals' from some people, or miss important things they are trying to tell us. It also explains why many nurses and other health care professionals find telephone interactions in the context of palliative and end of life care difficult. In that situation you are much more reliant on the words you use and how you say them. In addition you cannot see the person's body language to judge how he or she is reacting to the news. You need to rely on the individual's words and silences to gauge his or her response.

Touch in palliative and end of life care

Touch is an important aspect of non-verbal communication. In Activity 3.2, were Amy to have been present you might well have used touch to convey empathy. Touch is an important communication tool to use when undertaking complex and difficult conversations. Touch can convey what sometimes we would struggle to put meaningfully into words. However you must learn as a nurse to use touch when needed and appropriate for the individual, rather than having a blanket one-size-fits-all approach. There are many cultural and societal aspects that you need to recognise and respect when considering the use of touch. Using touch can support and enable communication, but it is crucial to remember it can also act as a blocking technique (see section on barriers to effective communication). As a nurse you may well be more comfortable with touch than some of the patients you support and care for. When you touch a patient/family member it should be because you believe it will help that person, not because the touch helps you feel more comfortable. It will also be important to remember that for some individuals the only touch they receive is when a carer is giving physical care.

This could be described as a technical form of touch, but as Clarke (2013) highlights, the way in which you touch a patient when undertaking even the simplest of care procedures such as taking blood pressure will communicate much about your attitudes and beliefs about your work and your patient. Your touch can help or hinder the building of the vital relationship between you and your patient. Often the most intimate aspects of personal physical care can create opportunities for very deep connections and meaningful communication, but only if our touch is thoughtful and based on kindness and compassion (see Chapter 2 for further discussions about touch, spirituality and holistic care).

Key facilitative skills to support communication in palliative and end of life care

The basic principle that underpins all interactions with a patient who is facing the end of life, or with a family member of theirs or a close friend, is for you to find out the patient's areas of concern. You will then use this information to focus on the patient's needs rather than focusing on your own. There are a number of facilitative skills that support and enable this approach. Table 3.2 discusses these and the context for their use.

Key facilitative skills (Goldberg et al. 1993; Zimmerman et al. 2003; Maguire et al. 1996)	Examples and contexts for use in palliative nursing practice
Open questions (OQ), open directive questions (ODQ)	*OQ*: 'How are you feeling?' As this question is very wide it enables the person to decide what to focus on and how much to tell you *ODQ*: 'Can you tell me about your pain?' This provides a more specific focus for the response but is still not overly prescriptive
Acknowledging (A) Reflecting (R) Paraphrasing (P)	*A* is a skill that allows us to demonstrate that we recognise the situation the person has shared with us *R* enables us to use patients' words back to them to show we have heard them, e.g. 'You felt really upset . . .' *P* allows us to use their words in a way which demonstrates our listening and comprehension: 'You found that time really painful' Often use of these skills will encourage patients to tell us more about their feelings because we have demonstrated our interest
Checking/clarifying (C/Cl)	*C/Cl* can help you to identify if you are getting the gist of what you are being told accurately
Summarising (S)	*S* can help us to demonstrate we have been listening attentively: 'So you said that things have been going quite well but you have been concerned about your mother and also the increase in your neck pain, especially in the mornings.' We can also ask patients/family members to *S*, as a way to check out what they know or have taken in. 'Can you tell me what you have been told so far about your illness?' N.B.: This is a better way of putting this question than: 'What can you remember about what they told you about your illness?'

Table 3.2: Key facilitative skills and their use in palliative and end of life care

You can practise the facilitative skills in Table 3.2 and over time they will become embedded within your nursing practice. However there may be times when you feel out of your depth; when you are unable to answer a question or that you do not know how to address a concern expressed by a patient or family member. This might be when a patient or relative asks you a difficult question outright.

Scenario

Imagine you are nursing Mrs Jill Cox, who has advanced multisystems atrophy and is unable to communicate verbally. Her brother Philip comes to see her. He meets you in the corridor and asks you, 'Is Jill dying?'

Activity 3.3	*Critical thinking*

Using the information in Table 3.2, consider what key facilitative skills you would use in this situation. Use the following points to guide your discussion:

- What open and open direct questions might you ask Philip?
- What would you say to acknowledge how Philip is feeling at this time?
- How would you reflect back to Philip what he is feeling?

An outline answer is given at the end of this chapter.

At times like the situation in Activity 3.3 you may not know the answer to the question. You may refer on to another colleague or seek guidance from a colleague and then speak with the person again. If you do not know the answer it is acceptable to say: 'I'm sorry, Philip, but I don't know the answer to your question.' If you express empathy and concern for him, and offer alternative help to acquire an answer you will have recognised the concern expressed and addressed that. It may have taken Philip a huge amount of courage to express his concern. The crucial thing is not to ignore his concern, or worse still, to dismiss it.

The role of silence in communication in palliative and end of life care

Additional to the key skills already mentioned, the use of silence is known to enable and facilitate communication (Eide et al. 2004). Pauses, particularly in the context of breaking bad news or other difficult conversations, help your patients by giving them time to think through what has already been said. Remember, when people are ill, frail or in distress, it may take longer for them to process information anyway. Pauses will aid patients to consider if they wish to ask a question, or not; if they can trust you, or not; and to consider how they are feeling about what has already been said. Although it may seem silent to you, there will usually be much 'internal dialogue' going on in the mind of the patient. Of course silence can sometimes help you too as it gives you a moment to think, or 'catch your breath'. Maintaining a pause in the conversation is often very difficult; your natural instinct might be to speak and 'fill the void'. Enabling a pause often leads the patient to talk more. However, if the pause becomes uncomfortable for patients, try to find a way to encourage them to speak. Try to avoid filling the silence simply to avoid your own discomfort, but in order to enable them to express themselves. Perhaps you could ask them gently if they can tell you what they are thinking. Be aware though that sometimes thoughts can be too difficult to put into words and if patients do not want to talk, then respect that. It may be that you revisit this with them at a later date.

The use of cues and educated guesses in palliative and end of life care

A cue is when a person gives a hint, verbal or non-verbal, that suggests an underlying emotion. A cue provides you with an opportunity to explore and clarify what the patient has alluded to in the cue (Del Piccolo et al. 2006). If you are actively listening and responding appropriately to the presented cues then the patient is far more likely to open up and tell you more about the situation, fears and concerns. A sigh, a frown or a half-expressed thought may all be cues; for example, a tailed-off sentence: 'Lately I've been wondering . . .'. When patients use cues, this is an opportunity for you to use the key facilitative skills to explore with them their concerns and to provide them with information or advice or simply the opportunity to talk.

Educated guesses are used to try to interpret from what has happened or what the person has already told you, and to demonstrate sensitive listening. Educated guesses should always be offered tentatively. You do not want to assume that you know what the patient is thinking or feeling, or that you are putting words into their mouth. Educated guesses are often prefaced by a phrase such as 'It sounds as if . . .' or 'It seems like that might . . .'. Consider these two statements made by a nurse when a patient disclosed that, as a teenager, he had looked after his dying mother:

* 'That must have been very difficult for you.'
* 'It sounds like that might have been really hard for you.'

The first statement assumes that it could not have been anything other than very difficult to do this and it is likely therefore that the patient will agree with this. In the second statement you can sense the nurse is not assuming anything. In reality the patient may have been pleased to care for his mother, and may not have felt that it had been hard. The second statement enables him to say, 'Yes, it was really tough . . .' or 'I loved her, so although it wasn't easy . . .'. This may then lead to further information being disclosed which may help us to offer appropriate care in the future.

Case study

Paul

Paul is 44, married to Lisa, and living in a small terraced house in the village where he was born and has spent all of his life. Paul and Lisa have two children, who are both still at primary school. Paul has recently been diagnosed with advanced carcinoma of the pancreas, for which no curative options are available. He has had to stop work due to his disease, while Lisa is still working and juggling that with managing the children and home. You are working in primary care and, with your mentor, have been asked to visit Paul to assess his current and future needs.

When you arrive at the house Paul is alone. He tells you that Lisa is at work and that she collects their daughters from school on the way home and should be back soon. Paul invites you in and seems pleased to see you, although he is quite quiet at first. After a few minutes of casual conversation, he suddenly says, 'Do you think it will be long?'

Activity 3.4   *Critical thinking*

Consider Paul's case study above. How might you use some of the specific skills already discussed in this chapter to help find out what concerns and issues Paul may be worrying about?

An outline answer is given at the end of this chapter.

Activity 3.4 will have highlighted the importance of using skilled communication to support the assessment of a patient and his needs. It would be easy to dismiss Paul's concerns and undertake an assessment that overlooks these. You cannot assume what is uppermost in Paul's mind, e.g. financial concerns, spiritual concerns. The important thing is that you assess rather than assume.

Presence in palliative and end of life care

Your role in this part of a patient's life may be for just a few hours or for many months. Palliative and end of life care can occur in any setting, e.g. critical care unit, hospice or care home. The foundations of palliative care have been discussed in Chapters 1 and 2, together with issues around disease trajectories and the impact of these on care at end of life. Many skills, encompassing both 'the science' of nursing, e.g. pain management, and 'the art' of nursing, e.g. communication, are needed to provide compassionate care which maintains dignity and upholds autonomy in the face of increasing dependence and significant uncertainty. The care you provide will not only impact on the person who is dying but can have a major influence on the coping and bereavement of the family members, and therefore their future health and well-being.

The Francis Report (2013) into failings at the Mid Staffordshire NHS Foundation Trust identified a lack of compassion, at all levels within the trust, as a contributing factor to the neglect patients experienced. Nouwen (1982, p121) says compassion *asks us to go where it hurts, to enter into the places of pain, to share in brokenness, fear, confusion and anguish . . . compassion means full immersion in the condition of being human.* You might find this quote quite challenging; immersing yourself in someone else's pain and fear can be quite daunting. Developing your own *emotional resilience* and *emotional intelligence* will support you to deliver compassionate care and look after your own emotional well-being. In 2012 the Chief Nursing Officer identified compassion as one of the 'six Cs' (Commissioning Board Chief Nursing Officer and DH Chief Nursing Adviser 2012). Here compassion is encompassed with care: *compassion is how care is given through relationships based on empathy, respect and dignity – it can also be described as intelligent kindness, and is central to how people perceive their care.* This is, perhaps, a more accessible definition and places compassion in terms of communication and the therapeutic relationship you develop with your patients.

In palliative and end of life care communication and demonstrating compassion are not solely focused on verbal communication. Nouwen (1982) discusses the ministry of presence and how being with someone can, of itself, be a powerful and useful therapeutic and nursing intervention. Presence is a way of 'being' with a patient, encompassing behaviours that express caring and compassion. These include being sensitive and aware of the person and his or her needs, being attentive and focusing on the patient and his or her needs and connecting with the patient as a person (Covington 2003). In some situations you will not always be required to do or even to say anything; your presence, and the time you spend with a patient, is a form of communication in its own right and can be used as a successful nursing intervention. 'Being with' patients reaffirms to them that you value them and you are there for them; your presence may reassure them during a difficult procedure; your presence may support them to make a difficult decision (Covington 2003). Presence and 'being with' a patient focuses on the very heart of your relationship with your patient. It encompasses compassion, spirituality and person-centred care (see Chapter 2 for further information on spirituality and holistic care).

Activity 3.5   *Reflection*

Reflecting back on your clinical experience to date, think of a situation when you have witnessed a nurse, or other health care professional, using presence as a therapeutic and nursing intervention. Consider the following points:

- Could you identify when presence was used? What indicated this to you?
- How did the nurse demonstrate 'presence'?
- How did this support the nurse to engage with the patient on an interpersonal and spiritual level?
- What was the effect of this on the patient?
- What was the effect of this on the nurse?

The article by Wilson (2008) listed in the further reading section will provide you with further information to use in this activity.

As this activity is based on your own observations, there is no outline answer at the end of this chapter.

Activity 3.5 will have enabled you to consider presence and how it is used in palliative and end of life care as an effective communication method. You should not always assume, however, that at times of distress or when they are close to death, patients value having family members, other loved ones or a member of staff close by. Nouwen (1982) also suggests that for some, at particular times, absence can be as useful or necessary as presence. Knowing which approach to use relies on you having developed a positive therapeutic relationship with your patient, and his or her family or carer.

Barriers to effective communication in palliative care

Barriers to communication can exist either on the part of the patient/family member or the health care professional. Potential barriers to communication can take many forms, e.g. sensory impairment. You can use simple strategies, ensuring patients have their glasses on, and hearing aid in place and switched on. These will make a significant difference to their hearing and thus comprehension of any conversations that take place. Even those who are not obviously deaf may have some hearing deficit. Most people use lip reading to a degree, even though we may not be aware of it, and so consideration of your position and the person being able to see your face when you speak is also important. Patients with a neurological condition, e.g. Parkinson's disease, may lose their ability to use facial expressions to display emotion. Patients may be frightened to ask questions about their future – they may not want to hear the answer.

You may also put up your own barriers to communication by avoiding eye contact with patients, engaging them in 'small talk' or avoiding answering their questions (Maguire et al. 1996). To ensure effective and positive communication between you and your patients it is important that you recognise and understand the potential barriers that may be present, both in your patients and yourself. Gaining an insight into why your patients, and you, might create barriers will also promote patient-centred communication. In addition, recognising why you might 'block' communication will support the development of your emotional intelligence.

Two useful frameworks have been developed to support health care professionals in recognising why patients and health care professionals may put up barriers to communication. These can be remembered by the acronyms FEARS (fears, environment, attitudes, responses, skills) and FIBS (fears, inadequate skills, beliefs, support) (Tables 3.3 and 3.4). FEARS is used for potential patient barriers and FIBS is used for possible barriers present in you and other health care professionals.

FEARS element	Manifestation
Fears	Being judged as ungrateful; being stigmatised; crying/breaking down; burdening/causing distress to the health professional
Environment	Lack of privacy; person present or absent who needs to be/not be there with me
Attitudes	This person does not have time to listen to me, or it is not this person's job to talk about this; my concerns are not important; I should be able to cope with this; my family would not want me to talk about this

(Continued)

(Continued)

FEARS element	Manifestation
Responses (from health care professionals)	Distanced or disengaged; relevant questions were not asked of me; being touched when I need my own space
Skills	I cannot find the right words/have not sufficient command of language/do not understand enough to know what to ask; literacy levels; mental capacity issues

Table 3.3: FEARS: potential patient barriers to communication

FIBS element	Manifestation
Fears	Causing upset or harm; emotional responses; saying 'the wrong thing'; being asked difficult questions; taking too much time
Inadequate skills	Lack of assessment skills for psychological issues and concerns as well as physical ones; inability to integrate physical and non-physical agendas together into a full holistic review
Beliefs	Emotional problems are inevitable in serious/life-threatening illnesses; nothing can be done about them so it is pointless to bring up issues we 'cannot solve'; it is 'someone else's role to do this'
Support	Lack of support for the patient if problems are identified; feeling professionally unsupported; team conflicts

Table 3.4: FIBS: possible barriers in health care professionals

Activity 3.6 — *Reflection*

Reflecting back on your clinical practice, think of a situation where you found communication with a patient or relative difficult or challenging. Using both the FEARS and FIBS framework, consider what patient barriers may have impacted on the interaction and recognise what may have inhibited your ability to communicate effectively.

As this activity is based on your own observations, there is no outline answer at the end of this chapter.

Considering your own practice in relation to the above barriers should help you to be more aware of them in the future and to be able to address them in a constructive way.

There is significant evidence that people find it helpful to discuss their fears and concerns. There is not always an expectation or need for 'an answer'. However the barriers you identified in Activity 3.6

as impacting on your ability to communicate with people in difficult situations may prevent you from 'walking on dangerous ground'. Your concerns may prevent you from offering the patient the opportunity to talk. This in turn may lead to your patient's concerns and needs not being expressed or met. You may not always be able to prevent some of the barriers within yourself; however, the more self-aware you are, the more likely you are to work actively to address these barriers. Similarly, if you can be mindful of the types of issues which can hinder communication from the patient/carer perspective you may be able to use your own skills to mitigate against these. Skilful and empathic assessment to find out the worries and concerns the person is really experiencing and seeing things from that person's angle will of itself be beneficial, even if you cannot 'offer an easy solution'.

Complex communication in palliative and end of life care

Tuffrey-Wijne and McEnhill (2008) have noted the particular difficulties that caring for someone with a learning disability at end of life can pose. As a nurse you need to be aware of the complexities around truth telling and decision making. You will need to seek appropriate support to be able to offer the best possible opportunity for your patient to make his or her own decisions, or to have as much involvement as possible. Read (2006) reminds us that for family members the idea of the person with the learning disability having that degree of autonomy can be very hard and we have a responsibility to support family members who may already have suffered multiple losses in relation to this person.

Case study

Pauline

Pauline is 53. She has Down's syndrome and early Alzheimer's disease, characterised by an increasingly impaired memory and unusual restlessness. She lives in a small care home with three other residents and she seems happy there. Pauline's father died of a heart attack whilst he was in hospital recovering from minor abdominal surgery. Although she was very upset at the time Pauline seems to have coped well since and rarely mentions her dad. Her mother Susan visits her regularly and her two older brothers help Susan to take Pauline out at least once or twice a month, which she enjoys. Pauline attends a day centre and has a busy social life with her friends, particularly going to music events.

Pauline was diagnosed with type 2 diabetes two years ago. She has been admitted to hospital twice in the past six months because of recurrent chest infections. On her last admission she required two courses of intravenous antibiotics to eradicate the infection. This caused her great distress as she could not easily get up and around. She has said several times that she 'never wants to go back in hospital ever again, not even if I dies'.

The care home staff are all very fond of Pauline. She has been in their care for almost a year. She is a warm and friendly woman who loves fun and laughter. The staff have expressed concern to the GP

continued ...

> *about Pauline saying she does not want to go into hospital again if she needs treatment. They have tried to discuss this issue with Susan but she is adamant that Pauline must be readmitted if necessary. Susan refuses to discuss or even mention the matter with Pauline.*
>
> *Things come to a head when a new senior carer starts working at the care home. She tries to talk with Susan about Pauline's expressed wishes not to return to hospital. Susan becomes very angry and says that if the staff do not do as she asks she will sue the care home as they have no right to discuss things with Pauline as she, Susan, is Pauline's mother.*

Activity 3.7 — *Decision making*

You are accompanying the community nurse (Valerie) who is offering support to the care home team and helping to monitor Pauline's diabetes for the primary health care team. Pauline and Valerie have known each other for two years and have built up a good relationship. Pauline always refers to 'Valerie the vampire', and although you know she does not enjoy having blood tests done she has never refused them, as she says it helps her be able to have some sweeties sometimes. The care home phone and ask for help in talking with Susan.

Using the information in this chapter, consider the following:

- What potential barriers to communication is Susan displaying?
- What key facilitative communication skills could you use to explore these with Susan?
- Who might you consider including in any conversations?

An outline answer is given at the end of this chapter.

Activity 3.7 will have allowed you to relate some of the key principles of communication to a case study, in addition to considering effective communication in this case study, as well as issues around whether Pauline has capacity to make decisions for herself. Issues of consent in palliative and end of life care are discussed further in Chapter 8. Given the complexity of this situation Susan will need a significant amount of support throughout. The relationship that you make as a nurse with her is deeply important to being able to offer that support. The balance between upholding Pauline's rights and Susan's may cause tension and difficulties. In these kinds of situation the person often 'has an inkling' of the truth of the situation and is looking to us to confirm the reality rather than the news being a 'bolt out of the blue'. It is important to remember that confidence is much harder to regain once lost, and that all the team may be mistrusted once one team member is considered to be dishonest.

In situations where a child or young person is very ill, similar issues can arise and once again communication is at the centre of ensuring person-centred care. Review the case study below and then consider the questions that follow.

Case study

Jake

Jacqui is a staff nurse in a specialist plastic surgery unit. She has worked in this speciality for three years, having completed her preceptorship and consolidated her key skills in a general surgical ward for one year post NMC registration. She is keen to remain in this speciality and further her career.

She is on duty when a 15-year-old young man (Jake) is admitted, following a sudden and unexpected seizure which led to ambulance transfer from school to the Accident and Emergency department of the hospital. Jake has a previous history of malignant melanoma, which was first diagnosed 18 months ago. He has had two operations for this condition. Jacqui has not cared for Jake before, as his previous admissions were to the paediatric ward within the unit.

Jake is drowsy much of the time following admission and has severe headaches, nausea and vomiting. As the index of suspicion, or in other words the risk, that he may have developed metastatic cerebral disease is high, an emergency CT scan is ordered. On the day of the scan and so that Jake can receive medication for symptom control, Jacqui escorts him to the department for the scan. Jake remains very drowsy and is scarcely even speaking. Although Jacqui thinks he is aware that she is there, she is less sure that he remembers her from yesterday.

When the scan is performed it is clear that Jake has two large lesions within his brain. Jacqui feels very sad for Jake, his parents and his brother. She knows that it is now unlikely that Jake will live to full adulthood, although until scan results have been received it will be unclear what the next steps will be in offering treatment, care and support.

The entire procedure takes some time and Jake has been away from the ward now for two hours in total. When Jake is back on the ward and in bed he suddenly asks Jacqui, 'Did you see my scan? Could you see anything?' Jacqui is surprised by his question, in that he had not spoken at all until that moment, and she had thought him to be almost asleep. She does not know how to respond, although she does not want to lie to him. After a pause she replies, 'Yes, Jake, I did see the scan'. After another, even longer pause, Jake says, 'But I don't suppose you understood it, did you?'

Activity 3.8   *Critical thinking*

Using the information and the knowledge you have gained in reading this chapter, consider the following points:

- What information might you have wanted to ask/find out before taking Jake for his scan?
- What key facilitative communication skills could Jacqui use in this situation?
- What potential barriers to communication could Jacqui use in this situation?
- What might be the consequences of Jacqui not telling Jake the truth?
- Why do you think Jake may have replied as he did?

An outline answer is given at the end of this chapter.

The case study in Activity 3.8 has the potential to be particularly challenging; you may have included some of these challenges in your answers to the questions posed. Not only did Jacqui have to consider key aspects of communication, she also had to recognise the legal issues of open dialogue with a minor without a parent present (see Chapter 8 for further information regarding this).

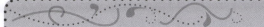

Chapter summary

Within this chapter we have considered the various helps and hindrances to effective communication in the context of palliative and end of life care. The value of a therapeutic relationship has been the thread throughout, together with the acknowledgement of the emotional cost to you as a nurse of investing in such relationships with people facing loss and death. By using the skills discussed and being present and mindful in your interactions you will help not only your patients and those close to them, but also yourself to become richer and more rounded, both as a person and as a practitioner.

Activities: brief outline answers

Activity 3.2: Communication

This is a common scenario that you will meet in practice. Issues you might have wanted to consider in advance include:

- Had anyone explained to Amy that there might not be any warning of Peter's death and that it might not be possible for her to be present if something happened suddenly?
- Did Peter's notes contain information regarding any underlying health issues that Amy had?
- Did the notes give details of other family members or friends that you could contact (with Amy's permission) to be with her after you had broken the news of Peter's death?

Aspects you might have included were that you would find it more difficult to speak to Amy over the phone than face to face, because you would not find it easy to gauge her responses to you without the benefit of her body language. You would not know in advance if she was alone or had any family member or friend present. You would need to pay special attention to your tone as this would convey your compassion and empathy with Amy.

Activity 3.3: Critical thinking

- Open question: 'What has prompted you to ask this question?' Open direct question: 'Has something changed in Jill's condition that makes you think this?'
- 'That's a difficult question to ask. You must be quite worried about Jill.'
- 'I can see you find this difficult to talk about. Would you like to go somewhere quiet where we can discuss this?'

Activity 3.4: Critical thinking

In this kind of conversation your tone and body language will be crucial in conveying your willingness to enter into this topic if Paul wants to.

- Clarifying the time available for the conversation may be a helpful starting point for both of you. It will be difficult for him to 'open up' if he knows his child will be coming home in the next few minutes, or if he expects that you have only five minutes to spend with him. This is an approach that some practitioners find difficult, but in most care contexts patients are used to an unspoken timeframe of five to ten minutes, so hearing that you have more than this to offer could be very positive and create an openness and equality in the relationship from the outset.

- In addressing Paul's question it will be essential first to clarify what he means by 'Will it be long?' He might mean long until the disease progresses or until he dies – but he might mean until the family return. The use of very gentle reflection and echoing his words ' . . . be long until . . . ?' will offer him the chance to tell you what he means by that question, or indeed to decide he does not want the answer and therefore he may change the subject.

- Using open questions such as 'How are things for you at present?', or 'What are the most important issues for you right now?' will enable Paul to choose what to focus on, and may lead to disclosure.

Activity 3.7: Decision making

Things you might usefully have included in your answer are as follows:

- Susan might present the following barriers to communication. F (fears): she might be frightened she will cry and that she will burden the staff in the care home. A (attitudes): that she should be able to cope with this. S (skills): Susan may feel that she does not understand enough about Pauline's health to be involved in a discussion like this. In addition Susan may wish to protect Pauline.

- Acknowledging how Susan is feeling about this situation will help validate her feelings. The use of open and open direct questions will allow you to explore in more detail why Susan is reluctant to discuss future care needs with Pauline. Reflecting and paraphrasing back to Susan will encourage her, with your support, to explore her feelings behind her decision.

- Others you will need to involve include the GP, care home staff, and additionally the Community Learning Disability Team, who may help to offer advice and support. If necessary a referral to the Independent Mental Capacity Advocacy service can also be made.

Activity 3.8: Critical thinking

Key aspects and issues in this situation relate to both Jake's pre-existing knowledge and insight into his illness.

- It would be useful to find out what information Jake had previously been given and what he understood from that, as well as what information his parents are happy for him to have, particularly as they were not present at the time he asked the questions. Knowing what Jake's parents know and understand and the level of openness there is between them all about the disease and the future is fundamental, not only to effective communication, but also to offering supportive family-focused care.

- Jacqui could have used both open and open direct questions to find out why Jake had asked this question. Doing this would have allowed her to explore Jake's thoughts and feelings in more detail. Reflecting back and clarifying information would have ensured Jacqui understood what it was that Jake was asking. Jacqui used silence to allow Jake time to consider his first question and decide whether or not he was ready to follow this up with a further question.

- Jacqui could have presented the following barriers. F (fear): she might have been frightened to discuss this further with Jake; she might not have wanted to upset him. I (inadequate skills): Jacqui may not feel she has the necessary skills to discuss this with Jake; his age could be a contributing factor.

- If Jacqui had not told the truth then it seems very likely that Jake would have lost faith in her as a nurse. Even if he thought she was speaking the truth to begin with, he might well realise later that she had lied. Jake's family might also have found the telling of the lie very difficult to cope with.

- Jake's response may have been because he genuinely thought that Jacqui might not have the skills to understand the scan. However it could be that her expression told him the truth, and he did not need the words to confirm it. Another possibility is that Jake may have asked the question and then realised he did not want to hear the answer, and so he tried to deflect Jacqui from telling him. An alternative reason for him replying thus is that he may have been trying to spare Jacqui's feelings. He might have felt sorry for having asked her this difficult question, as patients sometimes do.

Further reading

Baughan, J. and Smith, A. (2013) *Compassion, Caring and Communication: Skills for Nursing Practice.* Harlow: Pearson.

This text explores the interconnectedness of three core components of excellence in nursing care.

Kabat Zinn, J. (2011) *Mindfulness for Beginners: Reclaiming the Present Moment and Your Life.* Boulder, CO: Sounds True.

This text provides an introduction to mindfulness, a practice derived from Buddhist teachings.

Wilson, M.H. (2008) 'There's just something about Ron': one nurse's healing presence amidst failing hearts. *Journal of Holistic Nursing,* 26 (4): 303–307.

Useful website

http://dyingmatters.org

This website focuses on raising awareness about dying, death and bereavement. There are useful resources about how to talk to people about death and dying.

Chapter 4
Exploring loss, grief and bereavement

Jane Nicol

NMC Standards for Pre-registration Nursing Education

This chapter will address the following competencies:

Domain 2: Communication and interpersonal skills

3. All nurses must use the full range of communication methods, including verbal, non-verbal and written, to acquire, interpret and record their knowledge and understanding of people's needs. They must be aware of their own values and beliefs and the impact this may have on their communication with others. They must take account of the many different ways in which people communicate and how these may be influenced by ill health, disability and other factors, and be able to recognise and respond effectively when a person finds it hard to communicate.

Domain 3: Nursing practice and decision making

4. All nurses must ascertain and respond to the physical, social and psychosocial needs of people, groups and communities. They must then plan, deliver and evaluate safe, competent, person-centred care in partnership with them, paying special attention to changing health needs during different life stages, including progressive illness and death, loss and bereavement.

Domain 4: Leadership, management and team working

4. All nurses must be self-aware and recognise how their own values, principles and assumptions may affect their practice. They must maintain their own personal and professional development, learning from experience, through supervision, feedback, reflection and evaluation.

NMC Essential Skills Clusters

This chapter will address the following:

Cluster: Care, compassion and communication

3. People can trust the newly registered graduate nurse to respect them as individuals and strive to help them to preserve their dignity at all times.

continued ...

By the first progression point

1. Demonstrate respect for diversity and individual preference, valuing differences regardless of personal view.

By entry to the register

4. Acts professionally to ensure that personal judgements, prejudices, values, attitudes and beliefs do not compromise care.

4. People can trust the newly registered graduate nurse to engage with them and their family or carer within their cultural environments in an acceptant and antidiscriminatory manner free from harassment and exploitation.

By the first progression point

1. Demonstrates an understanding of how culture, religion, spiritual beliefs, gender and sexuality can impact on illness and disability.

By entry to the register

5. Is acceptant of differing cultural traditions, beliefs, UK legal frameworks and professional ethics when planning care with people and their families and carers.

Chapter aims

After reading this chapter you will be able to:

- consider your role in providing care for those experiencing loss, grief and bereavement;
- explain models of loss and bereavement and use these to support patients, their families and carers;
- recognise differing cultural perspectives and the impact of these on nursing care of those facing loss, death and bereavement;
- support the bereaved at the end of life and care after death.

Introduction

Life is loss, grief, growth . . . a universal experience of cycles and circles:
we must grieve to let go, to grow, and to make future attachments.
(Humphrey and Zimpfer 2008, p12)

Loss, grief and bereavement are about more than just death and dying. Life is about loss, loss is integral to our lives and we experience loss throughout the journey of our life. The loss of our first tooth, our children leaving home, when we retire – whilst these losses can provide a person with the opportunity to grow, this is not always the case. Take, for example, people diagnosed with dementia. Here the decline in their cognitive function affects their ability to interact with their family and friends. For the person, family and friends there is a profound sense of loss, and bereavement, long before death: loss of the life lived, loss of the person and loss of the life still to be lived. Indeed death might ultimately be a welcome relief. People requiring palliative and end of life care, and their carer, family and friends, will have experienced many losses, from diagnosis onwards, and will continue to do so until death.

Recognising how you respond to loss, the factors that influence this, possessing a good knowledge about the theoretical concepts of loss, grief and bereavement, recognising the impact of these and using effective strategies to support those in your care will enable you to deliver sensitive, person-centred palliative and end of life care. To support you in your ability to care for this group of people, and their carers and families, this chapter will develop your knowledge in relation to loss, grief and bereavement. In order to do this the chapter will support you in exploring your thoughts and feelings regarding loss, grief and bereavement. It will also examine the theoretical concepts of loss, grief and bereavement, recognising cultural perspectives, and will provide you with some useful strategies to support those in your care.

Exploring loss

Loss is defined as the state of being deprived of or being without something one has had, or a detriment or disadvantage from failure to keep, have, or get. Grief is the pain and suffering experienced after loss; mourning is a period of time during which signs of grief are shown; and bereavement is the reaction to the loss of a close relationship.
(Humphrey and Zimpfer 2008, p3)

Loss, grief and bereavement are inextricably linked together, with each eliciting an emotional response, and this emotional chain commences with the loss of something, someone or some place. As such, loss can be categorised in the following ways (Humphrey and Zimpfer 2008; White et al. 2010):

- Loss of a relationship – this can be a very significant loss and may result from a break-up with a boy/girlfriend, divorce, moving to another area.
- Loss of an aspect of oneself – this can be physiological, such as loss of function due to cerebro-vascular accident (CVA) or loss of body part due to surgery. It can also be psychological, for example, a person's enjoyment of life due to depression, or a change in personality due to traumatic brain injury. The loss can also be of your independence either through illness or being punished in prison for committing a crime.
- Loss of an external object – this can be any object that a person values, whether a smart phone, a childhood toy or family heirloom. The loss of the object is not just financial value, but there is a sense of loss of history and family heritage. Some loss can be of sentimental significance, like a ring given to you by your mother.
- Loss of a familiar environment – this can relate to moving house, moving from primary to secondary school or being admitted into hospital. As strange as it may sound, loss of familiar environment can be experienced when you go away on holiday. For example, my seven-year-old daughter, on arrival in Christchurch, New Zealand, after a 36-hour flight, turned round

as we were walking to the airport terminal building and commented that she did not like it here and wanted us to go back home.

- Developmental loss – this type of loss is a natural part of a person's growth, and is often not recognised. It can include moving from carefree childhood to a more responsible adolescence.

Figure 4.1 is an example of a timeline identifying types of loss and the secondary losses experienced.

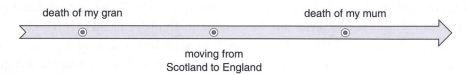

Figure 4.1: Example losses.

- Death of my gran – loss of a significant relationship and secondary loss of a familiar environment.
- Moving from Scotland to England – loss of significant relationships, loss of external object (I had to sell my flat) and loss of familiar environment (change in employment) and secondary developmental loss.
- Death of my mum – loss of significant relationship and secondary developmental loss.

The above timeline allows you to see that loss is part of the fabric of life. Some losses offer you new opportunities and other losses, such as the death of a loved one, you find harder to accept.

Undertaking Activity 4.1 will support you in developing your understanding of the losses experienced by people receiving palliative and end of life care. It is important to highlight the fact that each loss is perceived differently, which means there is an element of subjectivity when we consider the ideas of loss, grief and bereavement.

Activity 4.1   *Reflection*

This exercise will assist you to explore the concept of loss, as experienced by people diagnosed and living with a life-threatening condition.

On your own or with a group of your colleagues, work through the following exercise. If you are working in a group you will need to allocate a person to read out the story.

First write down the following:

- your five most prized possessions (material things)
- your five most favourite activities
- your five most valuable body parts

- the five values that are most important to you
- the five individual people whom you love the most.

Now as you read through this story, or have it read to you, cross out as many items on your list, from any category, as instructed. You must try and imagine how you might feel like while crossing off the items and what it may mean for you not having that item/person/ value any more.

Imagine it is a lovely spring day – you know the kind, one of the first days when the snow has melted and the flowers are blooming, the temperatures are comfortable and the birds are singing. You are successful and happy with your life. You step into the shower anxious to get on with the day. While you wash yourself you discover a small lump on your neck and another in your breast.

Cross out two items.

Probably swollen glands from your recent cold, you think. You ignore the lumps and go on with your life. Two and a half weeks later the lumps are still there.

Cross out two items.

Probably cold returning – you've been busy, not resting. You've had cystic breasts in the past, you rationalise, and life goes on; but something keeps nagging at you so you make an appointment to see your doctor.

Cross out one item.

The doctor, after examining you, refers you to the breast cancer specialist team at your local hospital. An ultrasound, mammogram and image-guided core biopsy are carried out. You are told: 'Your results will be available in five days; depending on these we will schedule you for surgery.' Friends try to reassure you that it will be OK.

Cross out three items.

Your results confirm it: you have breast cancer. You are waiting to go down to theatre. You and your surgeon have decided to opt for breast-conserving surgery but you have also decided to go ahead with a mastectomy if needed.

Cross out two items.

You pull yourself up through the fog in the recovery room and feel the mass of bandages on your chest. Your worst fears have been confirmed!

Cross out four items.

You recover from your surgery and have a course of radiotherapy just in case.

Cross out two items.

Slowly you recover your strength and life returns to normal, almost. It is spring again, two years later. You have a cold. You ignore it as usual but it doesn't go away; one morning, to your surprise, you find it difficult to breathe.

continued ...

Cross out two items.

Lung metastasis: you feel your world turn upside down again. That wonderful defence mechanism of denial must be let go. You begin chemotherapy and are very sick, weak and angry. You lash out at your family, doctors and friends. You want to live but you cannot eat.

Cross out two items.

One morning you do not have enough energy to sit in a chair; the doctor tells you that the chemotherapy is not working and he wants to stop it.

Cross out three items.

It seems like life goes on around you in slow motion. Days and nights blur. How odd, you think, staring at your bony hand, as your body deteriorates, your spirit seems to be withdrawing also. You wonder if it's the pain medication or if it's the first taste of death, but you do not have the energy to ask anyone.

Cross out the last two items.

Now answer, or discuss, the following questions:

- What was it like to cross items off your list?
- What did you cross off first?
- What did you cross off last?
- Was it harder to cross off items as you went through the story?
- Did you cross off all your items or did you stop?

The above exercise is adapted from Matzo et al. (2003) and incorporates NICE (2004) guidelines.

Brief answers to all activities are given at the end of the chapter, unless otherwise indicated. This activity is based on your own observations, so there is no outline answer given.

In Activity 4.1 the items you placed on your list, the order in which you crossed items off and your responses to losing your items will be unique to you. They will be influenced by many things: your age, your gender, your spiritual or religious beliefs and your cultural background. This will be the same for people diagnosed and living with a life-threatening condition; they too will have unique responses to their losses based on their individual circumstances. As individuals, with our unique perspectives on life, we can never completely *understand* how another person is feeling. Recognising your emotional responses to loss, as in Activity 4.1, will better equip you to recognise your own emotions, and the emotions of others, enabling you to empathise with those in your care. As emphasised in Activity 4.1, people living with a life-threatening condition experience loss throughout their illness, from diagnosis to end of life care. These losses can result in feelings of grief and bereavement; therefore their responses to loss may relate to known models or theories of bereavement. Whilst this chapter focuses on loss in relation to death and dying, the principles of this can be applied to loss as it occurs in different settings and with various conditions. An understanding of the relationship between loss, grief and bereavement will support you in caring for people living with terminal illness or other illnesses that impact on their daily life. Indeed, how individuals respond to loss has been a topic of much debate and study.

Models of grief and bereavement

Not all palliative and end of life care takes place in a specialist palliative care setting, therefore as a nurse it is likely that there will come a time when you are faced with the death of a person in your care. You are then witness to the grief, and bereavement, of the person's family, carers and friends. In some way, due to the nature of your relationship with those in your care, you share the loss with the family, carers and friends. The grief that follows loss should be recognised as a natural response to loss and there is no one way to grieve. How often have you heard someone who is bereaved say 'I'll get over it' or 'I know I can work through this'? Alternatively you might hear a person say 'Surely she should be over it by now' about someone who is bereaved. Grief does not just disappear; it stays with the person throughout that individual's life. Your role is to provide support that allows the bereaved person to find a place for his or her grief and the deceased while enabling the person to carry on *living*. Death and dying can provoke strong emotional responses in us (see Chapter 1). Being self-aware, recognising and managing the emotions you experience in relation to loss, grief and bereavement will enable you to develop positive therapeutic relationships with those in your care (see Chapter 2 and Nicol 2011).

Over the past century or so many models and theories have attempted to explain and rationalise people's experiences of grief in response to a significant loss and subsequent change in their life. These models have discussed grief and bereavement from a variety of perspectives, such as the stages of grief, the process of grief and attachment and loss. Understanding these models will provide you with knowledge of the broad theoretical concepts. Applying these to those in your care will assist you to support those who are bereaved. When applying these models to people in your care, you should be aware of the influence their values, beliefs and culture has on them and how these shape their experience of grief and bereavement. Doing this will enable you to deliver person-centred culturally sensitive care that recognises and celebrates the diverse population in the UK. Chapter 5 discusses aspects of culture and caring in a multicultural way. There is not scope in this book to discuss all models and theories; further reading is mentioned at the end of the chapter. However, it is pertinent that we discuss the seminal works and some of the more recent models and theories.

Sigmund Freud: *Mourning and Melancholia*

Sigmund Freud, in his seminal work *Mourning and Melancholia* (1917), was perhaps the first person to put forward an explanation of grief and bereavement. Written against the backdrop of the First World War, Freud recognised the attachment people had to the deceased and that in grief people who are bereaved give up not only the deceased but also a part of themselves. He referred to the emotion felt during bereavement as 'mourning', with the bereaved person's emotional energy still invested in, and attached to, the deceased (Payne 2004). In his discussions Freud stated the requirement for the bereaved to disengage from what has been lost, withdraw energy, and subsequently invest this energy in new attachments. In doing this he recognised the many layers of attachment and the secondary losses that are present. The suggestion by Freud would mean that the bereaved may not continue with their life until they have successfully detached themselves emotionally from the deceased. This has attracted criticism as most people believe they can carry on with their life without completely detaching themselves. The important thing to say is that people learn to manage their emotions and now and again can put them to one side (compartmentalise them) while concentrating on the here and now of life.

Kübler-Ross: *On Death and Dying*

Elisabeth Kübler-Ross's work *On Death and Dying* (1973) is perhaps the most widely recognised work in the area of loss, grief and bereavement. It was published at a time when death and dying were taboo subjects. Her study was based on the belief that most people feared dying, *not* death, with people believing it to be a lonely, impersonal experience. Her aim was to understand this process better and so support those who are dying in coming to terms with their own mortality. Kübler-Ross interviewed over 200 people who were dying, encouraging them to discuss their thoughts and feelings about their own dying and death. From these interviews she identified five stages people that are dying experience: denial, anger, bargaining, depression and acceptance. The stages are seen as coping mechanisms, defence strategies or ways of maintaining hope that can overlap, exist at the same time and are human responses to dying. Therefore, it should be recognised that those who are dying may not experience all of these stages or experience them in that order.

Over time Kübler-Ross's theory has been adopted to cover those who are bereaved as well as those who are dying. This adoption, however, has been challenged. Research has identified that, when death occurred through natural causes, i.e. the death was anticipated, acceptance rather than disbelief (denial) was the most prevalent emotion felt by the bereaved. However in the case of sudden death, disbelief (denial) was found to be the most frequently experienced emotion (Maciejewski et al. 2007). This is also relevant in palliative and end of life care. Even when death is expected, many patients with organ failure, e.g. heart failure, can die suddenly due to an acute event such as a myocardial infarction.

Activity 4.2   *Critical thinking*

Take the time to consider some of the issues that you might be faced with when applying Kübler-Ross's work to those who are bereaved.

An outline answer is given at the end of this chapter.

Despite the challenges identified above and in Activity 4.2 in relation to applying Kübler-Ross's model to the bereaved, it should be recognised that Kübler-Ross gave a voice to those who felt isolated, providing them with an opportunity to teach others about their experience.

Klass, Silverman and Nickman: *Continuing Bonds*

The model proposed by Klass et al. (1996) called into question previous perceptions (Freud 1917) that stated grief was something to work through and a detachment from the deceased made, in other words to 'break the bonds' with the deceased. Klass et al. (1996) stated that bereavement should be considered as a cognitive and emotional process that takes place in the context of a person's life, of which the bereaved person is part. Their work proposed that maintaining bonds with the deceased was normal in mourning and could contribute to successful adaptation of the bereavement. However they do not prescribe that bonds should be maintained; indeed it is recognised that for some, maintaining bonds with the deceased can be counterproductive (Field 2006). For example, some people may feel compelled to continue a relationship with the deceased by going to put flowers on the grave and maintaining its surroundings. Widowed people may find it hard to remarry; these aspects can be argued as being counterproductive. For others, maintaining a continuing bond with the deceased preserves memories. Walter (1996) suggests that there are two types of bonds: private and public. Private bonds are those that are kept private through thoughts and feelings; these can include sensing the presence of the dead, spiritual relationships or symbolic places and things. Public bonds are those that others are aware of and the deceased can become an ancestor, spoken about and remembered by family and friends. Goodhead (2010) analysed memorials to deceased loved ones on the St Christopher's Hospice 'Tree of Life'. His analysis found that continuing bonds, declaring an ongoing loving relationship between the bereaved and deceased, featured in up to 69.6 per cent of the memorials written. It is true to suggest that when you help the bereaved 'deal' with the public bonds, it will help them to manage their private bonds more effectively.

Stroebe and Schut: the Dual Process Model

The Dual Process Model introduced new thinking in relation to loss, grief and bereavement. Rather than focusing solely on 'grief work', it emphasised the role that other coping strategies play in helping the bereaved (Stroebe and Schut 1995). Stroebe and Schut explain that grieving is a dynamic process where the bereaved oscillate between different coping behaviours (everyday life experiences) termed 'loss orientation' and 'restoration orientation'. Loss orientation focuses on the loss of the person who has died and includes grief work, e.g. talking about the loss, crying. Restoration orientation incorporates addressing the additional losses faced by the bereaved, such as returning to work or managing household finances. This oscillation allows the bereaved person to take time off from the pain of grief, which can be overwhelming, enabling the bereaved to cope with day-to-day life and the changes in it.

The Dual Process Model emphasises that both loss orientation and restoration orientation are necessary to allow the bereaved to adjust to their new future. However the authors recognise that the emphasis on loss orientation and restoration orientation will vary from person to person depending on the circumstances of the death and the personality, gender, age and cultural background of the bereaved. Stroebe and Schut state that this model can also be used to identify complicated or unresolved grief, allowing appropriate therapeutic interventions to be put in place. This can be used to support bereavement counselling by identifying which part of the model the person spends most of their time in. Strategies can then be implemented to support the person to manage grief and bereavement more positively.

Applying the models to your care

Gaining knowledge and developing an understanding of these models will assist you to identify where a person is in his or her grief. Read through the case study below and consider which models of loss, grief and bereavement are relevant.

Case study

In the days following the death of her mother, despite having her family around, Julie felt very alone. She couldn't possibly believe that anyone else was feeling as desolate as she was, yet she knew this was selfish. What about her dad? How was he going to cope? He had been so strong; did he have any strength left? Everyone who knew her mum was hurting – her dad, her brother and his family, her sister and her family, not to mention her own husband and children.

As soon as she heard that her mum had died the tears began, and for the moment wouldn't stop. She had known her mum was dying but still she felt angry – should she have been there? She had last visited her parents a week before her mum died; she lived 300 miles away, worked and had a young family to look after. She could see then that her mum was worse; she wasn't eating, couldn't stand and was so tired. Through her tears Julie also felt a sense of relief – relief that her mum's 'battle', because that is what it had been, was over and she was at peace. The pain we are feeling, she thought, was nothing compared to the pain her mum experienced over the last year of her life.

Back home at her dad's with her brother and sister, Julie stood in the room where her mum had died. It was empty – the hospital bed, commode and wheelchair were all gone. It still smelt of her mum and Julie found this comforting, although her tears began to flow again.

Julie found that helping to organise her mum's funeral gave her purpose, something to do that took her mind off the pain she was feeling. She decided she would like to read a poem at her mum's funeral. She was advised against this; however this only increased her determination to do it – this was going to be her tribute to her mum, and it was. With all her family around, Julie sometimes felt overwhelmed by everyone's emotions and a sense of claustrophobia crept in. She needed to be on her own, remembering her mum in her own way. During these times she lay on her bed listening to music or went out for a walk, whatever the weather.

The funeral over, back home and back to work, Julie had the day-to-day concerns of work and family to occupy her mind. Yet her mum was always there, and Julie's tears were never far away. She went for walks on her own, talking to her mum about the day's events, telling her what had happened and crying. The nights were the worst: she couldn't sleep, or if she did, she would wake up crying and lie there quietly until the morning. Although her husband comforted her during the night, she still felt lonely. Then in the morning, she just wanted to pull the duvet up over her head and stay there, but she thought about her dad. He was getting up every day to an empty house. If he could do it, then so could she. Julie threw herself into her work; it was a welcome distraction from the sense of loss that had crept into her life, her new life where everything had changed. Yet when she looked out the window she saw the world was the same. How could this be? Couldn't others see that everything was different?

The first year was the hardest. Family celebrations, birthdays and anniversaries came and went without her mum being there, yet there were also glimpses of happiness, memories and stories shared, photographs laughed over. Was it possible that life could be good again, different but good? Could she allow herself to be happy? On the first anniversary of her mum's death Julie took out her mum's engagement ring from the drawer where she had kept it since her mum had died. She decided the time was right to wear it, and she wears it on her wedding finger along with her own engagement and wedding ring, as a constant reminder of her mum. Time passed. It's been over two years now. Julie still thinks of her mum every day and talks to her, and although her pain is easing, what she is left with is a sense of sadness that she knows will stay with her. She finds this comforting; her mum will be with her forever: she is part of her, part of her children and a constant presence in her family's life.

It is evident in the case study that a number of models of loss, grief and bereavement are applicable to Julie. In the early days Julie feels anger at the death of her mother despite knowing that it was inevitable. Here you could identify Julie as experiencing one of the stages of dying, as discussed by Kübler-Ross (1973). It is also possible to identify elements of the Dual Process Model (Stroebe and Schut 1999), with Julie focusing on restoration orientation by helping to organise her mother's funeral and later throwing herself back into her work. Loss orientation is also evident when her emotions resurface and she cries. Perhaps the most significant model to be evident is Klass et al.'s (1996) Continuing Bonds. Julie has maintained a significant bond with her mum, which is also extended to other family members. Her bond has both a physical aspect, the wearing of her mum's engagement ring (private and public bond), and an emotional aspect, talking to her mum (private bond) and talking about her mum with family (public). These bonds provide comfort to Julie and allow her to find a way for her mother still to be part of her, and her family's, life.

Activity 4.3   *Reflection*

Using the information above, reflect back on your previous practice or placement experience. Which models of loss and bereavement have you seen displayed in patients, carers, family or staff? You may find it helpful to read the article by Greenstreet (2004) to develop your understanding of these models. The full reference for this article is listed in the further reading section at the end of this chapter.

As this activity is based on your own observations, there is no outline answer at the end of this chapter.

Both the case study above and Activity 4.3 will have enabled you to explore the various responses people have when faced with the death of a loved one. Having a good understanding of the models and how they apply to your clinical practice will assist you in recognising how people who are bereaved respond. It will also enable you to discuss loss, grief and bereavement with bereaved people, reassuring them that their response is natural.

It is important that you understand that you may end up using different aspects from different models and use them together to help support the patient and the bereaved. With practice you will develop skills to select the most useful 'bits' from a range of different models for your own use. For example, where there is denial you may allow more time for the bereaved to come to terms with their loss. And where there is anger, you may want to acknowledge it and then empathise as a starting point in helping the bereaved.

As discussed in this chapter, people's responses to loss, grief and bereavement are individual and personal to them. This requires you to be sensitive to this and to adapt your care and support accordingly. This is also the case when considering people with additional care needs such as people living with a learning disability. Increasingly people living with a learning disability are living longer. This means they are more likely to experience one or more significant bereavements in their lifetime, e.g. the death of a parent. For people living with a learning disability their loss may be compounded by the fact that the deceased was their primary carer.

Research summary: bereavement and learning disability

In 2002 MacHale and Carey carried out an investigation into the effects of bereavement on the mental health and challenging behaviour of adults living with a learning disability. They had a sample size of 20 adults living with a learning disability who had experienced bereavement of a primary carer in the last two years and a matched control group. Of the 20 who had experienced the death of a primary carer, 90 per cent were living with the carer until time of death, and as a result, 40 per cent had to move out of the family home. Their study also found that all the participants attended the funeral and 70 per cent were known to keep a memento of the deceased and 65 per cent visited the grave of the deceased on a regular basis.

When focusing on mental health and challenging behaviour the results of their study indicated statistical significance in relation to:

- psychiatric disturbance – neurotic disorder and organic condition;
- challenging behaviour – irritability, lethargy and hyperactivity.

MacHale and Carey recognise the limitations of their study: the number of participants was small and the information was gathered from carers, not the participants. Given the high percentage of participants who experienced secondary loss, such as having to leave their family home, it was not possible to separate out the impact of the primary (death of the carer) and secondary losses. However, their study does demonstrate that bereavement has a significant impact on those living with a learning disability, with resulting implications for nursing care.

The impact of concurrent losses, loss of primary care giver and family home, was a theme identified by Blackman in 2008. Blackman (2008) focused on the development of a bereavement needs assessment tool (BNAT) that would help to identify the bereavement needs of people living with a learning disability (see page 78 for an application of this to clinical practice). By focusing on the holistic needs of a person, the tool can be used to clarify specific bereavement needs. The aim of the tool is to provide appropriate person-centred support. One of the effects of this could be a reduction in challenging behaviour being displayed by the bereaved person living with a learning disability.

Case study

Jenny

Jenny is a 45-year-old woman with Down's syndrome. She lives with her mother and father; they are both retired and are Jenny's primary carers. As well as having Down's syndrome Jenny is partially deaf; she communicates using speech and Makaton but finds communicating with more than one person at a time hard. Jenny is loving and friendly. She enjoys watching films and going for walks with her dad. Jenny attends a day centre twice a week, where her favourite activity is helping in the kitchen. Both Jenny's parents go to church regularly; Jenny attends with them and enjoys the support and friendship that the congregation provides.

Last week, while Jenny was at the day centre, her father collapsed at home. He was admitted to hospital and following investigations was found to have had an extensive CVA. He has been in hospital since then, and has not regained consciousness. Jenny and her mum visit every day. Since her dad's illness Jenny has not been attending the day centre; she does not want to go back in case the same thing happens to her mum. Jenny has been told her dad is very ill, and that he may die. Three days ago they received a phone call to say that her dad has had a further CVA and could they come to the hospital immediately. Shortly after their arrival on the ward Jenny's dad died. Jenny did not want to be with her dad when he died as she found the situation rather frightening. Instead she sat with a member of the nursing team while her mum was with her dad. Jenny did not want to see her dad after he had died, but she did give the funeral directors her favourite teddy bear to put in her dad's coffin.

Jenny attended her dad's funeral and cremation with her mum and other family members as well as friends from their local community and church. Jenny is able to understand that she will not see her dad again; this frightens her and she is worried about this happening to her mum.

Undertaking this assessment will allow you to assess a person living with a learning disability and her level of understanding about her bereavement (Table 4.1). This will allow you to identify areas for concern. Recognising and identifying these potential problems will allow you to discuss a plan of care that addresses these.

Area to consider	Questions to ask	Application to Jenny and her care
Emotional responses	• Does this individual recognise his/her own emotions? • Can he/she express these emotions?	Jenny is able to recognise her own emotions; she knows when she is happy/sad Jenny can express how she is feeling either verbally or via Makaton
Cognitive understanding	• How do the people around the person respond to his/her expression of emotion? • Does this individual have an understanding of the concept of death? • Does this person have an understanding of the permanence of the new situation? • If the death was expected, did the person have an understanding of this?	Jenny's mum is very attentive and focused on Jenny's well-being Jenny has been told her dad has died; however she is finding it difficult to understand that she will not see him again Jenny had been told that her dad was very ill and that he might die
Social responses	• Was the person informed of the expected death? • Has the individual been informed of the death? • Who informed the person and how?	Jenny had been told by her mum that her dad was very ill and that he might die
Social impact	• What significance has this loss had on the person's familial network? • What significance has this loss had on the person's social network? • What has the impact of the loss been on other members of the familial/social network? • What changes in role have to be negotiated? • What quality of support is available?	Jenny has lost one of her primary care givers; she spent a lot of time with her dad out walking Jenny has not returned to the day centre since the day her dad became unwell The fact that Jenny does not want to return to the day centre will reduce her social interaction and increase her dependence on her mum

Area to consider	Questions to ask	Application to Jenny and her care
Physical	• What has the impact been on the person's physical health?	There has been no obvious impact on Jenny's physical health; however she did take regular walks with her dad. This was her main form of exercise. It might be necessary to think about how to maintain Jenny's level of activity
Lifestyle	• Has this loss meant a move from the family home? • Has this meant more than one move? • Has this person experienced other significant losses? • What other lifestyle changes has this created?	Jenny and her mum are still able to stay in the family home Jenny misses going out for walks with her dad
Continuing the relationship with the deceased	• Did the person see the deceased shortly before he/she died? • Did the person attend the funeral? • Does this person have access to photos and mementos of the deceased? • Is this person able to visit the grave, if there is one? • Is this person able to reminisce with others who knew the deceased?	Jenny saw her dad the day before he died and she was able to attend his funeral There are lots of photos of Jenny's dad in the family home Jenny is able to talk to her mum about her dad, though they both get upset
Changes in functioning	• Has this person's ability to communicate with others been affected by this loss? • Has this person lost any skills since this bereavement?	Jenny is still able to communicate with those around her; she has not lost any of these skills

(Continued)

(Continued)

Area to consider	Questions to ask	Application to Jenny and her care
Spiritual	• In what ways has this bereavement affected this person's religious or other spiritual beliefs? • If this person was part of a local religious community/congregation, is he/she still able to keep those links? • What meaning has the person attached to this loss?	Jenny and her mum have been supported by their local church community This is the one place Jenny feels able to visit at the moment Jenny understands her dad has died and that she will not see him again – this frightens her
Changes in identity	• To what extent has the loss affected the individual's self-concept and self-esteem?	Jenny has lost some confidence; she is worried that if she returns to the day centre her mum will become unwell

Table 4.1: Application of Blackman (2008) bereavement needs assessment tool to Jenny

As you can see from the case scenario and the assessment in Table 4.1, there are several areas that should be addressed as part of Jenny's, and her mum's, bereavement support. Jenny has stopped attending the day centre, she no longer goes for walks and she has lost some confidence. To support Jenny, and her mum, you would commence a care plan allowing you to address these issues, for example, supporting Jenny to return to the day centre. You might begin by discussing with Jenny what her fears are and getting her to visit the day centre with her mum. In addressing this issue you may also begin to increase Jenny's confidence. It is important that Jenny maintains her exercise levels, not just for the physical benefits but also for the psychological ones; therefore you could suggest that Jenny and her mum start going for walks together. Jenny could show her mum her favourite walks that she went on with her dad. This would support Jenny to maintain both private and public bonds with her dad.

Religious considerations in loss, grief and bereavement

Within palliative and end of life care part of the aim of holistic care is to reduce a person's anxiety about death. Assisting a person to find meaning to his or her life and to integrate that meaning to his or her life can support a person preparing for death (Chung 2000). Meaning can be found through religion, which helps individuals to be at peace with themselves. To support this, the National Institute for Health and Clinical Excellence's quality standards for end of life care for adults (NICE 2011) recognises the need for a person's religion to be addressed as part of holistic care at end of life:

- Standard 6: people approaching the end of life are offered spiritual and religious support appropriate to their needs and preferences;
- Standard 12: the body of a person who has died is cared for in a culturally sensitive and digni-fied manner. In addition, standard 12 needs to recognise that people who are dying and who have died should be cared for in accordance with their religious teachings.

One thing is certain: whatever the religious orientation, people will be touched by death, and it is not certain that they will be touched in the same way. Therefore, how they grieve and mourn will be strongly influenced by their religious orientation, with most religions having developed rituals related to grief and mourning (Clements et al. 2003). The UK population is changing, bringing with it a more religiously diverse demographic, and you need to respond to this by providing person-centred care that is sensitive to people's religious needs. This section only focuses on religious aspects: you can read more about cultural care in Chapter 5.

Case study

Ali is 65 years old and has been living with chronic kidney disease since he was 25. He is a devout Muslim and lives with his wife Nabila. They have three children: two daughters, Nyla and Sanna, and a son, Tariq. Ali's children and their families all live close by and are very supportive. Ali's faith is very important to him and it has helped to keep him strong throughout his life.

Recently Ali has been told that his second kidney transplant is failing and, following a conversa-tion with his family, Ali has decided not to have any more dialysis. Ali and his family know that by refusing further dialysis his condition will deteriorate and he will eventually die. Ali has accepted this, but is worried about the impact of this on his family. Ali has stated that he would like to remain in his own home, and if possible die there, and this is an arrangement all his family are in agreement with.

For Muslims, whose religion is Islam, illness and disease may be regarded as a test from Allah. Therefore it is expected that the sick person should be stoical and pray to Allah to alleviate pain and suffering (Cheraghi et al. 2005). This means that the view of Muslims towards illness includes the idea of receiving illness and death with patience and prayers. Muslims believe that death is not the cessation of this life, but that the person's spirit is eternal and lives on. For many Muslims health and illness are part of the continuum of being, with prayer providing salvation in both health and sickness. One important point to emphasise is that this may be different from how you or your family approach death and dying issues. When caring for a patient with differing values and beliefs, maybe like Ali, it is crucial that you remind yourself to respect their prefer-ences and wishes, even if you do not agree with them.

Activity 4.4   *Evidence-based practice and research*

Two days ago Ali's condition deteriorated quite quickly. The Primary Care Team, with Ali's family, made the decision to commence the Liverpool Care Pathway for the Dying Person. Ali is being nursed at home by his family with support from the District Nursing Team. You are working with the District Nurse (DN) and visit Ali and his family twice a day to offer support.

Task 1

In order to respect Ali's and his family's Islamic faith, what care do you need to take into consideration during his final days?

One afternoon, whilst visiting another patient, the DN you are working with receives a phone call from Ali's son. He says his dad's condition is worsening; his breathing is becoming more laboured. The DN explains to Tariq that she will be with them as soon as she can. When you arrive at Ali's house you are met by his son, who says his dad has died.

Task 2

In order to respect Ali's and his family's Islamic faith, what do you need to take into consideration now that he has died?

To help you answer these questions use the following references:

Cheraghi, M.A., Payne, S. and Mahvash, S. (2005) Spiritual aspects of end-of-life care for Muslim patients: experiences from Iran. *International Journal of Palliative Nursing*, 11 (9): 468–474.

Gatrad, R. and Sheikh, A. (2002) Palliative care for Muslims and issues after death. *International Journal of Palliative Nursing*, 8 (12): 594–597.

An outline answer is given at the end of this chapter.

Activity 4.4 has focused on the religious aspects of Ali's care before and after death. As well as recognising these, it is important that you utilise effective communication skills and demonstrate non-judgemental care, e.g. active listening, reflecting and accepting the family's thoughts and feelings. Following Ali's death the family will adhere to a period of mourning; this is generally for three days and is known as *hidad*. It is likely that the women and men will mourn separately. During this period of mourning the Qur'an will be recited. During *hidad* it is customary for friends and family to visit the bereaved and offer their condolences. Ali's family will not prepare any food; this will be prepared by their friends, relatives and other members of their community. Nabila, Ali's widow, will observe a longer period of mourning (*iddah*) which lasts for four months and ten days.

This case study and activity focus specifically on Ali and his individual needs. The knowledge you have gained from reading this chapter will enable you to apply these principles to your nursing practice in palliative and end of life care, taking into consideration people's religious, spiritual and other preferences.

Care after death

For many the concept of a 'good death' includes not just the care given up to the time of death but also the care given to the deceased after death (Pattison 2008). The care given after death encompasses what has, in nursing, been traditionally referred to as 'last offices'. The term 'last offices' not only relate to nursing's military and religious roots but also to the Christian sacrament of 'last rites' (Quested and Rudge 2003). Care after death is the last caring act you as a nurse can perform for the deceased. It allows you to demonstrate your respect for the deceased and family. It allows you to 'close the chapter' in that you have cared for the patient during life and you will care for him or her after death (Kwan 2002). It is important, therefore, that when you perform care after death it is done in a sympathetic and sensitive manner (Nyatanga and de Vocht 2009). This encompasses being sensitive to any specific religious or cultural requirements and demonstrating respect for the deceased and the bereaved through compassionate care. Providing the bereaved with the opportunity to remember the deceased in a peaceful way, with catheters removed, hair brushed and clean night clothes, has the potential to help the bereaved take their first steps into their future life without the deceased.

Activity 4.5   *Reflection*

Using a model of reflection, e.g. Gibbs (1988), and the following questions as prompts, reflect back on a situation where you have performed care after death. If you have not performed care after death yourself, discuss these questions with your mentor/registered nurse:

- If appropriate, how were cultural and religious practices addressed/maintained during last offices?
- How were the privacy and dignity of the deceased maintained?
- Was there any aspect of performing last offices that you found particularly difficult? If yes, then why was this?
- Were there any aspects of performing last offices that you found particularly comforting? If yes, what were they?
- How did you demonstrate support for the bereaved?

Using a model of reflection will assist you to structure your reflection, ensuring that you stay focused on a specific topic. Using the questions listed will further increase your level of analysis of the situation, and this will develop your ability to analyse critically your own practice and that of colleagues.

As this activity is based on your own observations, there is no outline answer at the end of this chapter.

As you can see from Activity 4.5, when performing care after death, as well as caring for the deceased and the bereaved, it is important that you take care of yourself. To be able to perform care after death in a positive way you need to possess an understanding of the skills and emotional resilience you require to enable you to carry out this act (Nyatanga and de Vocht 2009). The importance of carrying out care after death properly includes:

- helping the bereaved to start life after death with positive memories of the deceased;
- helping the bereaved to view a calm and peaceful-looking image of their loved one;
- helping you raise awareness and understanding of your own perceptions and biases about death;
- helping you to be aware of your own response and reaction to death each time you perform care after death;
- helping you and the bereaved to 'close the chapter' with the deceased;
- helping to commit the deceased into a new beginning in future life.

Reflecting on these throughout your clinical practice will support you to develop the knowledge, skills and attributes required to perform care after death with maximum benefit for the deceased and bereaved and minimum anxiety to yourself.

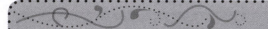

Chapter summary

This chapter has provided you with an overview of loss, grief and bereavement and its application to holistic care in palliative and end of life care. The concept of loss has been explored and models of grief and bereavement have been discussed and applied to a case scenario. This approach will support you in recognising the individuality of bereavement and how a person's grief changes over time and the importance of maintaining bonds with the deceased. Recognising the differing requirements of those with a learning disability when faced with loss, grief and bereavement has been explored and related to nursing practice. The importance of respecting and honouring a person's religious requirements at end of life has been discussed. The effect of sensitive care after death on the bereaved, and you as a nurse, has been recognised.

Activities: brief outline answers

Activity 4.2: Critical thinking

Having a fixed, linear idea of how a person will grieve could impact negatively on the type of post-bereavement care you provide. For example, when a bereaved person has accepted the death of the loved one early in the grieving process, this could be misinterpreted as complicated grief, with the offer of bereavement counselling seen as inappropriate. This could result in the bereaved person feeling that you are not listening to his or her needs, resulting in a loss of trust and a breakdown in the therapeutic relationship. This could subsequently prevent the bereaved person from seeking support from you in the future, if necessary.

Activity 4.4: Evidence-based practice and research

Task 1

- Support Ali's family to ensure that the local Iman is available.
- It is important, where possible, that the soles of Ali's feet face the Qiblah in Mecca (direction in the UK south-east); therefore Ali's bed should be moved to allow this to happen. If this is not possible, then it is permissible for Ali's face to be turned to the direction of the Qiblah.
- Friends and relatives should be allowed to gather round Ali.
- Privacy should be allowed as family members may wish to recite prayers; this will include the Declaration of Faith.

Task 2

- Once the death has been verified, Ali's body should be prepared in accordance with the wishes of his family.
- Ali's body should be treated in a gentle and dignified manner.
- If at all possible, only people of the same sex as the deceased should touch the body; therefore only males should touch Ali (where practical).
- After his death Ali's body should not be touched by a non-Muslim. Therefore it would be appropriate to ask permission first from the family and to wear gloves.
- Ali should not be left with his feet facing the Qiblah. Instead his body should be positioned to allow his face to be turned to the right and face the Qiblah.
- Ali's eyes should be closed and his body straightened out. This is done by flexing and straightening the elbows, shoulders, knees and hips, in the belief that it will prevent Ali's body from stiffening.
- Any excess fluid, blood or excrement can be cleaned from Ali's body, though his nails should not be cut. Ritual cleansing will be carried out as soon as possible by a male Muslim.
- Ali's body should remain covered at all times.
- Ensure that all documentation is completed in a timely manner. This reduces the likelihood of any delay in the funeral taking place; burials take place within 24 hours.

Further reading

Greenstreet, W. (2004) Why nurses need to understand the principles of bereavement theory. *British Journal of Nursing*, 13 (10): 590–593.

This article provides a review of the most well-known bereavement models.

Pattison, N. (2008) Care of patients who have died. *Nursing Standard*, 22 (28): 42–48.

This article outlines the steps involved in preparing the deceased after death, including religious considerations, legal and aftercare for the family,

Useful websites

www.dyingmatters.org

This is the website for the Dying Matters coalition; their aim is to raise awareness of, and change attitudes towards, death, dying and bereavement. Their site contains useful resources, for both health care professionals and those living with dying, on relevant topics relating to death and dying.

http://www.endoflifecare-intelligence.org.uk/home

This is the website for the National End of Life Care Programme. The aim of this programme is to improve end of life care for adults in England. However there is information on this site that is applicable to all people who are receiving palliative and end of life care.

Chapter 5
Exploring the impact of cultural issues in palliative and end of life care

Brian Nyatanga

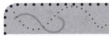

NMC Standards for Pre-registration Nursing Education

This chapter will address the following competencies:

Domain 1: Professional values

2. All nurses must practise in a holistic, non-judgemental, caring and sensitive manner that avoids assumptions; supports social inclusion; recognises and respects individual choice; and acknowledges diversity. Where necessary, they must challenge inequality, discrimination and exclusion from access to care.

Domain 2: Communication and interpersonal skills

1. All nurses must build partnerships and therapeutic relationships through safe, effective and non-discriminatory communication. They must take account of individual differences, capabilities and needs.

NMC Essential Skills Clusters

This chapter will address the following:

Cluster: Care, compassion and communication

3. People can trust a newly qualified graduate nurse to respect them as individuals and strive to help them preserve their dignity at all times.

First progression point

1. Demonstrates respect for diversity and individual preference, valuing differences, regardless of personal view

Entry to the register

4. Acts professionally to ensure that personal judgements, prejudices, values, attitudes and beliefs do not compromise care

4. People can trust a newly qualified graduate nurse to engage with them and their family or carers within their cultural environments in an acceptant and anti-discriminatory manner free from harassment and exploitation.

continued ...

   First progression point

1. Demonstrates an understanding of how culture, religion, spiritual beliefs, gender and sexuality can impact on illness and disability.

   Entry to the register

5. Is acceptant of differing cultural traditions, beliefs, UK legal frameworks and professional ethics when planning care with people and their families and carers.

6. Acts autonomously and proactively in promoting care environments that are culturally sensitive and free from discrimination, harassment and exploitation.

Chapter aims

After reading this chapter you will be able to:

- discuss the idea of culture and how it is transmitted from one generation to the next;
- explore possible modifications to culture as a result of living in a multicultural society;
- explore cultural differences and associated issues when caring for people receiving palliative and end of life care;
- explore the idea of multicultural society and the need for nurses to be culturally competent in their care for dying patients;
- discuss what type of knowledge and skills nurses need to become culturally competent in caring for diverse patient groups.

Introduction

In order to understand people and their identities, you need to understand their culture and its rituals. However, we do not all agree on what culture is. In order to increase your own understanding of culture, this chapter will start by discussing in more depth this lack of consensus. Attending to and being aware of cultural differences is one of the central aspects of the unique individualised care you provide at end of life. With different cultures come varying rituals to be observed during and after death. It is quite possible that patients you care for, who are dying, may experience similar symptoms, but the meaning attached to these may not always be the same. Therefore, any intervention offered by you and other health care professionals should recognise such cultural differences. This assertion conveys a serious challenge. It implies you should be able to recognise and understand all these differences and use this to provide person-centred care in palliative and end of life care. For you to be able to converse fully with all the different cultures means you have to be *culturally competent*. Today's Britain is a multicultural society, which means that, in addition to being culturally competent, nurses and other health care professionals are expected to be multiculturally competent in order to continue to provide truly individualised care. Therefore, the question here is: how can you and other health care professionals develop such knowledge and skills to care in multicultural communities? First, let us consider what culture is and what it means for different people.

Understanding culture

The word *culture* is often used in different ways and contexts, and at times is used to refer to race, skin colour and nationality. The term is also used in relation to work practices: the 'culture of care' at Mid Staffordshire hospital, the 'culture of phone hacking' by newspaper reporters, the 'culture of fiddling expenses' by Members of Parliament, the 'culture of using performance-enhancing drugs' in sport. These examples show that culture as a term is not easy to define or understand, and that it may not have a universal definition. However, this comment may be premature; Activity 5.1 will support you to explore what you understand culture to be.

Activity 5.1   *Reflection*

Write down what the term culture means to you. While you are doing this, can you also think how you came to understand culture in this way? For example, was it through reading books, newspapers, listening to the radio, social experiences of mixing with different people or watching television? Maybe it was influenced by discussions you had at home with family and friends.

Brief answers to all activities are given at the end of the chapter, unless otherwise indicated. This activity is based on your own observations, so there is no outline answer given.

In Activity 5.1 you may have sought to describe culture from a social perspective, which tends to be commonly used in the literature. From this social view, culture is considered to be what governs a group of people in how they live their lives: the attitudes, values and beliefs those people hold and share *as a group*. It is important to say you cannot actually see the beliefs and values people hold. This is where the behaviour of people towards something can tell you about their attitudes and subsequently their culture. For example, you would not be able to tell by looking at people whether they are Christian, vegetarian or racist unless you saw them at church or eating their meals, or discriminating against someone based on race. Such sharing of ideas is not at a physical level (e.g. sharing a vegetarian dish) but at a psychological level, because beliefs and values are similar. However, we often find that people with similar beliefs and values *may* also share physical aspects like skin colour, living space and geographical backgrounds. For example, people living in the same region may share similar values and beliefs about marriage, whilst student nurses working together may end up sharing some values about how to care for patients with compassion. For the nursing students you may want to suggest that they would have similar professional cultural values that guide their practice. The commonly used definition talks about culture being *a set of attitudes, values and beliefs shared by a group of people and [that] tend to govern their behaviour in society* (Matsumoto and Juang 2007).

Categories of culture

The above description falls under the *normative* category of cultures. As far back as 1992, Berry and others came up with different categories of culture (Table 5.1) as a way of showing some of the fine difference between the categories. Looking closely at Table 5.1, you will see that the categories tend to overlap. This shows how culture is intertwined into these different aspects of people's ways of life.

Type of culture	Description	Comment
Descriptive	Focuses on different activities or behaviours associated with a culture	Used to enhance understanding
Historical	Refers to the heritage and traditions associated with a group of people	Similar to genetic
Normative	Focuses on rules and norms associated with a culture	Commonly used with definitions
Psychological	Focuses on learning and problem solving in order to strengthen a culture	Rarely discussed, and ill understood
Structural	Focuses on societal and organisational structures of a cultural group	Often implied in the discussion
Genetic	Focuses on origins of a culture	Similar to historical

Table 5.1: Categories of culture, based on Berry et al. (1992)

You may be wondering how these characteristics differ from religion. Thinking in this way shows that you are beginning to grasp the finer points about culture and that they have strong connections with aspects found in religion, for those with a faith. However, the simple answer is that culture and religion are different.

Activity 5.2 — *Reflection*

Take some time to reflect on what you already know about religion and culture, and write down what you see as the main differences between the two entities.

As this activity is based on your own observations, there is no outline answer at the end of this chapter.

You might have found Activity 5.2 quite difficult as it can be challenging to try and separate these two entities. The way some people live can be influenced by both culture and religion. Both culture and religion are underpinned by beliefs and values that hold and guide the way people live their lives. You can begin to separate these two if you consider what people do to fulfil their cultural and religious needs. Religious people would probably pray, go to a place of worship or attend gatherings to share thoughts and prayers. Another way of separating these two is when we include people who do not have a religion (faith) to guide their lives. For example, atheists (people who do not believe in God) or those without any faith whatsoever still have a culture. However, the way in which they go about fulfilling their cultural needs would be through different ritualistic practices such as visiting the sea every year and not by going to church.

Understanding culture is necessary to understand yourself and others (in terms of beliefs and values) and your place in the world, or, in some cases, the world we would like to live in, and how this can be carried through or passed down to other generations. It is the natural responsibility of parents/guardians and elders in society to make sure that these cultural norms are transmitted from one generation to the next. The process of transmitting cultural norms to the next generation (enculturation) suggests that culture is something you are not born with but learn as you grow up. You learned your initial values and beliefs from your parents, the society you grew up in, the people you socialised and played with and went to school with. Enculturation is therefore important for the survival and continuation of generations and their identities. However this process can be interfered with when we live in a multicultural society.

Modification of culture

Natural transmission of culture from one generation to the next has often offered insurance that deeply held values and beliefs are carried forward in different communities and societies at large. For example, the stoicism or 'stiff upper lip' found among the British is still continuing despite exposure to different belief systems. The exposure to different cultural belief systems inevitably tends to modify the existing cultural norms found in enculturation, and it is true that the British upper lip may not now be as stiff as it was. Such modification is often referred to as acculturation, which suggests that different cultural groups may adapt their original views, values and beliefs following exposure to other cultures. Such exposure takes place in different ways and at different times. For example, education is often seen as the first and most fundamental modifier of values and belief systems (Nyatanga 2008a).

Education has the power to liberate minds and in some cases can lead a revolution against parental influences, if these are seen as restrictive or narrow. You may be wondering why people would end up modifying their cultural values and beliefs. There are two key reasons for this. First, it is possible that people modify their cultural beliefs in order to survive in their environment. For example, small groups of immigrants settling in the UK may have no choice but to modify in order to survive. They need to speak the language, communicate with health care professionals and engage with the etiquette of the host culture. Failure to do so might mean they remain at the periphery and therefore marginalised in society.

Scenario

Imagine you have a friend who still insists on hand-writing letters and posting them as he does not believe in using emails. He does not believe in having a mobile phone either, and still uses the landline telephone at home. Whilst he has valid reasons for not modifying his values about communication

continued ...

> *(e.g. to keep the postman in a job, and not become a victim of mobile phones), he may soon find that the world around him is changing with new technology and therefore he will be forced to modify if he wants to continue communicating with friends and his family.*

The second possible explanation may be that, once exposed to other cultures, individuals may like or prefer some of the new values, such as equality for women, and may modify their own beliefs accordingly. Acculturation is therefore a feature of multiculturalism. It is important that we acknowledge that there are both benefits and drawbacks to acculturation in a multicultural society.

Activity 5.3 — *Critical thinking*

Take some time now to think about what you already know about acculturation and make two separate lists:

- the benefits of acculturation when caring for patients receiving palliative care;
- what you see as negative aspects of acculturation when caring for patients receiving palliative care.

The benefits and negatives can be for the individual, group of individuals or society at large.

As this activity is based on your own observations, there is no outline answer at the end of this chapter.

In Activity 5.3 you may have seen that acculturation brings many benefits for the patient but also challenges for you as a health care professional. You could argue that acculturation brings about closer integration between different cultural groups. With integration comes a better understanding of each other's values and beliefs systems. When this happens, care delivered will most certainly meet the needs of the different patients we care for, and hopefully we can ensure an individualised death with dignity. When acculturation happens in palliative care, it can lead the need for cultural competence in the care we give to dying patients. When completing Activity 5.3 you may have recognised that you need to develop your cultural competence. Cultural competence will be discussed in more depth later in this chapter.

It is clear from the summary in Figure 5.1 that recognising acculturation and incorporating each aspect into your patient care at end of life will lead to a dignified death for your patients. It is important that we look at the bigger picture when we consider acculturation, but, most importantly, the impact of this on the patient. It is also clear from Table 5.2 that there are drawbacks of acculturation. Some are quite subtle, like loss of identity, while others are more apparent, such as overt peer pressure to behave or dress in a certain way. The point that needs making from this is that both benefits and drawbacks need closer integration if we are to achieve the best outcome (the best death) for dying patients.

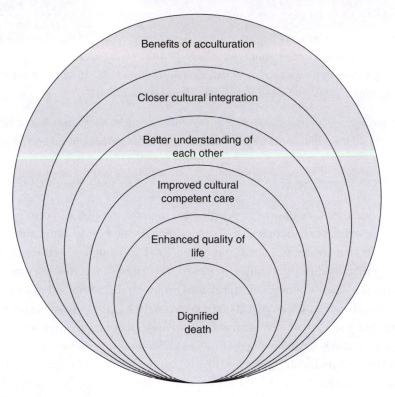

Figure 5.1: Benefits of acculturation.

	Drawbacks
	Threat to or loss of cultural identity
	Modifying to survive and possible resentment
	Challenges of multiple modifications
	Much harder on older generations, therefore may 'cling' to traditional values

Table 5.2: Drawbacks of acculturation

Case study

JP Junior, a 28-year-old single Afro-Caribbean man, migrates to the UK to take up a new job as a staff nurse in Worcestershire. This is his first time in the UK and he speaks relatively good English, achieving 7.5 on his International English Language Testing System test. He has one relative (an uncle) who lives in Dundee in Scotland. Although the decision to come to the UK is on the whole beneficial for his career and life, he has a few things to get used to. He needs to adjust quickly to the cold weather, since he arrived in September. The days are short and it gets dark around 5 o'clock. He needs to get used to the different food and the taste. JP will need to 'pick up' the language very quickly in order to be able to communicate effectively with patients and relatives. The art of communication has proved difficult

continued ...

even for the indigenous members of staff, therefore JP needs to work hard and train to be able to recognise cues, so critical in communication, and explore them. JP needs to understand the unofficial language often used colloquially by patients, relatives and even health care staff. All these aspects contribute to JP's ability to adapt, adjust and settle into a new cultural environment.

Socially, JP needs to understand the etiquette to socialise with others, make friends and maybe to find love. To achieve all this will take time, effort and resilience. Without the right support for JP, this transition may be quite uncomfortable and he may often feel homesick.

The case study demonstrates that most people who migrate to another country have to make adjustments. Adjustments help people like JP to survive in the new environment and also to appreciate difference in so many areas, such as way of life, food and language. However, when people have no choice but to modify, this can threaten their own identity. It is well documented that very often people from smaller or minor cultural groups resent modification and to an extent this may lead to intercultural conflict (Nyatanga 2008a). What might help resolve such conflict is for both groups (minor and major) to modify in an attempt to understand each other better. However, for the major culture this may mean having multiple modifications in response to each of the smaller or minor cultures in a multicultural society like Britain today. Another drawback concerns age: the longer the person has lived without exposure to other cultures, the harder it becomes to modify. The point to suggest here is that the older person's values and beliefs would also be deeply held, and therefore much harder to modify when compared to a younger person's.

One important and final point in this discussion is offered by O'Neil in 1995, cited by Nyatanga (2008a), that even after considerable acculturation, most cultures will revert to their original values and beliefs when it comes to births, marriages and death rituals. These events are seen as significant and in palliative care you tend to witness the death and dying rituals. Therefore it is crucially important that you also understand those original cultural values that existed before any acculturation took place. Once you start to understand, you can begin to believe in the idea of cultural competence.

Cultural competence

The need for cultural competence among health care professionals is well documented (Cortis 2004; McGee and Johnson 2007; Nyatanga 2008b), although it is not clear whether ideas of cultural competence fit well with the changing multicultural world of patients. The need for health care professionals to be culturally competent seems even greater now than before, with the idea being increasingly necessary in all settings, like the workplace, in politics and in social gatherings. The idea of cultural competence has been emphasised as part of a way we can increase the understanding of differences between cultures and thereby reduce potential disparities in care (Parekh Report 2000; Cortis 2004; Nyatanga 2008b).

Cultural competence has had numerous definitions and in health care systems it tends to focus on the ability of health care providers to deliver effective care for patients with diverse values, beliefs and behaviours. This definition goes some way towards clarifying what is needed to be culturally competent. However it does not go far enough, as it fails to include language differences and awareness. These can be an agent for increasing access to palliative care services by all patients and a powerful strategy to attract or encourage patients from black and minority ethnic (BME) communities to access services with confidence. This is an important outcome for caring in palliative care, not only for the patient but also for the whole family unit.

Activity 5.4   *Critical thinking*

What does cultural competence mean to you as a nurse caring for people in a multicultural society?

An outline answer is given at the end of this chapter.

The UK is a multicultural society; Activity 5.4 will have highlighted the many aspects of culture to take into consideration in your nursing practice. It is likely that in the future the UK will become increasingly multicultural due to population migration.

Migration

When writing my first book in 2001, I quoted 5.5 per cent of the UK population as BME and now the latest figures give it as 17.5 per cent (Office for National Statistics, UK Census 2011) (see weblink for the Office for National Statistics at the end of the chapter, where you can find out the cultural breakdown in your own region). It can be assumed that these numbers will continue to increase as the world becomes a much smaller place and people are free to migrate. Such an increase suggests that the UK is truly a multiracial and multiethnic society; therefore the needs of people when they are dying are bound to be as diverse as their cultural backgrounds. This diversity poses a challenge for you and other health care professionals. It demands that you become culturally competent when delivering palliative care to patients who are different from you.

It may be useful to start by going back into a brief history of migration to the UK by some BME groups. It is understood (Firth 2001) that the history of migration of ethnic populations to the UK is different for each group. Some came as families while others came as individuals looking for work. However, what was common was that, when factories closed and other jobs finished, many of the immigrants moved to East London, Birmingham and Bradford, where they have lived ever since. These towns have witnessed increasing poverty and premature death among this population group. The incompatibility of service provision and people's needs at end of life meant that most people died without proper care (Firth 2001). Although care may have been provided, it failed to reflect the individuality and uniqueness of dying people in terms of their cultural needs. Therefore, regardless of the high quality of care offered, it was not appropriate for some patients. It is like going to a top Michelin restaurant where they serve exquisite beef, lamb and chicken dishes, and every diner rates them highly. However, these dishes would not be ideal for a vegetarian diner, and therefore can be criticised for failing to meet the needs of this group.

The same argument applies to the palliative care services you provide for patients and whether these take into account the patient's cultural needs. Doing it this way will ensure that services are both suitable and acceptable for your patient. The other point to make is that cultural differences exist in the way people perceive health, illness, ways of coping, treatment, care and dying. Therefore to be culturally competent, you need to be aware of these differences and intervene appropriately. Cultural competence can be summarised in two broad ways – ability and knowledge – and explained thus:

- ability to interact effectively with and care for people of different cultures from your own;
- have knowledge-based skills to provide effective clinical care to patients from different ethnic or racial groups.

Benefits of cultural competence

Where services and care are provided based on cultural needs, they are likely to be acceptable to the patient and families. Think of the example of the restaurant given above, and that the exquisite dishes it serves must be appropriate to all diners.

It is likely that there will be an increase in the uptake of palliative care services if these are acceptable and also accessible. The other benefit points to the elimination of cultural disparities in care delivery. Because palliative care may not always give us a second chance, cultural competence can help us to get it right first time (NCPC 2012). However, if we were to 'flip the coin', we can easily see what the drawback might be of any service that is not culturally competent. It is important that we improve our communication with patients so that we can raise our awareness of their differing needs. Chapter 3 discusses aspects of communication and the skills needed when caring for patients who are dying.

However, it is more important that we can also be aware of ourselves and how we react and respond in the face of cultural difference. I am talking of being consciously aware of our own prejudices and biases, as the first step in liberating ourselves and how we care for people who are culturally different from us.

Activity 5.5   *Reflection*

This activity requires you to think back to a time when you were working in clinical practice and experienced or witnessed a patient's cultural needs not being assessed and met.

Write down what you think contributed to the lack of identification of the cultural needs of this patient. What was the impact, if any, on the patient and the health care professionals concerned?

As this activity is based on your own observations, there is no outline answer at the end of this chapter.

It is likely that some services are not designed to cater for cultural diversity and this can be a disadvantage for patients from BME groups. When BME patients' needs are not clearly identified, it follows that their needs will not be met. This may also mean they will not experience enhanced quality of life and their death may not be dignified. Health care service providers can improve their services by employing people from BME groups as part of the caring team, although this alone can create another problem, which is assuming that they understand everything about the BME patient. There are advantages, including sharing of information and knowledge about difference, while giving confidence to BME patients to access the service.

There is evidence (McGee and Johnson 2007; Nyatanga 2011) that in order to be culturally competent you need to have a number of attributes. There is debate as to whether these attributes can be developed at the same time, or that they develop one after the other and tend to build up to the expert level. Most of the evidence points to a sequential development starting with awareness, as shown in Figure 5.2. The suggestion is to view this set of attributes needed to be culturally competent as a set of building blocks (taxonomy), starting at the base and building up.

Awareness, as briefly discussed above, includes conscious awareness of self in the first instance in the face of difference and then being aware of the other person's value system and needs. After awareness, attitude about difference follows, and is based on our own beliefs about cultural difference. Attitudes can either be favourable or unfavourable towards cultural difference. Knowledge is thought to be a key, if not fundamental, attribute in cultural competence, as this helps carers to modify their attitude and behaviour towards cultural difference. Knowledge tends to 'tap in' to other wider aspects to do with human rights law, equality, professionalism and moral and ethical components of delivering palliative care. While this is happening, your own knowledge about yourself increases and your thoughts about cultural diversity become clearly defined. Finally, the skills necessary to deal with cultural diversity are thought to have developed sufficiently to be considered culturally competent.

It is important to discuss one other aspect that is necessary if we are going to be culturally competent – that is, the need to have cultural desire (Campinha-Bacote and Campinha-Bacote 1999) to develop all the above attributes effectively. Cultural desire is viewed as a social construct

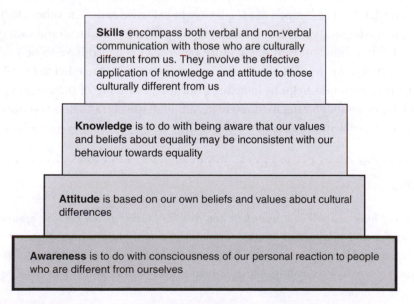

Figure 5.2: Building blocks of cultural competence.

which makes us have a natural inclination to engage in understanding cultural difference, and thereby pursue processes that lead to cultural competence. Campinha-Bacote (2002) describes characteristics of cultural desire as passion to engage with difference, commitment to achieve cultural competence and deep caring for the other person. In the end, when cultural competence occurs, it is something we no longer think about consciously, but tends to be second nature within us, based on our awareness, knowledge and skills to ensure cultural competence is effective. You could therefore amend Figure 5.2 by adding 'cultural desire' around all the attributes given. This would ensure that those who engage in cultural competence are serious and are not distracted by prejudice or stereotypes.

While the attributes in Figure 5.2 can be used as a useful guide for practice, there are challenges associated with them. For example, how would you know the minimum cultural desire necessary to engage fully with the process of cultural competence?

Activity 5.6   *Critical thinking*

Look again at the attributes in Figure 5.2. What are the challenges you might face in achieving or maintaining cultural competence in the area where you are studying?

An outline answer is given at the end of this chapter.

In Activity 5.6 you may have noted that there is no valid way of measuring or assessing cultural competence. You might have concluded that all these attributes are meaningless unless one has cultural desire to engage with this process. Cultural desire is seen a fundamental (Campinha-Bacote and Campinha-Bacote 1999) and is the 'glue' or commitment that binds all the other attributes together. You may also have thought about the challenge of measuring these attributes in order to say what level of competency is effective in palliative care. The other challenge worth highlighting in the implication of being culturally competent in a multicultural society is that you are not only being competent with one culture but in fact you also have to be multiculturally competent. You may have thought of language as a necessary aspect needed to be culturally competent. Linguistic awareness helps by increasing our understanding of the meaning of what the patient is telling us without having to translate it. Although use of translaters is common in palliative care, the only problem could be that some of the essence of meaning gets lost in translation.

Scenario

On a visit to China in 2009 on a study tour, you find the Chinese do not have an equivalent of the words palliative and hospice, and therefore it can be difficult to translate these terms into the main Chinese language, Mandarin, or the other 52 dialects. You realise that what can happen is mistranslation, leading to misunderstanding, and as a result patients may make decisions based on wrong or inaccurate information.

For palliative care professionals, mistranslation could lead to less dignity in death, if the patient's needs are not properly met. In some UK families translation is done by the younger generation, which can place a burden on them having to confirm bad news to their respected elders. It is therefore not surprising when the translation is deliberately distorted to avoid such a mental burden.

To go over the key point again here, the fact that most societies are multicultural suggests that being culturally competent also requires one to be multiculturally competent. Conversely, the impact of multiculturalism is a breakdown of traditional family configurations due to intercultural marriages and other cross-fertilisations (Matsumoto and Juang 2007). As this cross-fertilisation continues with acculturation increasing as well, it creates new challenges about culture and cultural groupings. By extension, this will pose challenges on the idea of cultural competence. It is therefore important that we ensure cultural competence is effective in order to provide culturally acceptable palliative care to all patients. While this is a reasonable aim to achieve, the way the cultural world is changing presents us with another problem, that of whether cultural competence might be achievable after all. Because the world is becoming an increasingly multicultural place, this has a tendency to distort or blur the cultural divides and boundaries that are currently present. Therefore, in addition to our current cultural competence, we need a third way of understanding the emerging nature of patients from these multicultural backgrounds.

Cultural competence in a world of multiculturalism

Everyone has an ethnic 'something' about them, and some people find themselves in the minority as a group when compared to other ethnic groups, therefore referred to as minority ethnic groups. Normally the colour of their skin and country of origin are used to differentiate their ethnic group (e.g. black British or white Irish minority ethnic). This can be neither right nor an accurate way to describe people of different ethnic backgrounds. When you consider how the future generation coming out of a multicultural society might present, some of the terms used at present will be redundant and therefore meaningless. For example, with new family configurations, future generations of patients may defy traditional conceptions of culture and ethnicity, and therefore classifications used today may no longer be helpful in terms of what they tell us about difference among people.

This may mean a gradual blurring or loss of clear ethnic and cultural boundaries on which the current idea of cultural competence is based. The point is that, although cultural competence may remain a noble aspiration for health care professionals to achieve, this should be placed in the context of the changing cultural world (Nyatanga 2011). It is from such changes that future assessments, service provision and palliative care may require different approaches to understand emerging cultural groups in order to continue to achieve cultural competence.

One of the first, and also most important, things we do in order to understand the needs of our patients is to make an initial assessment on admission to our caseload. We collect a lot of data, including medical history and also ethnic and cultural background. This information is used for different purposes, including formulating the patient's plan of care. Figure 5.3 is a typical example of some of the options patients are asked to choose from, and you might have come across similar forms during your clinical placements. In the next activity you can think about the importance of asking patients about their cultural background during nursing assessments.

Because of the complexity of accurately capturing patients' cultural backgrounds, there is a need to review how we assess patients' needs. Most writers, including Kai et al. (2007) and Nyatanga (2008a, 2011), now advocate focusing on the patient as a person and not as a cultural being. Rather than keeping on developing new tools for assessing patients from different cultural groups, it may work out better for both sides if student nurses and newly qualified staff are helped to feel confident enough to ask patients what matters most to them and how they can best help them.

For example, you could ask: What brings you here? What is bothering you the most? Can you help me understand you and your needs? Do you have any rituals/practices that I should be aware of in order to help you with your illness while you are with us on this ward/unit?

What is important here is to think of what it is we are trying to understand by ascertaining ethnic/cultural background. Also, what do we intend to do with the information? Apart from acquiring statistical information about the different types (cultural groups) of patients accessing and receiving care, other reasons are dubious. Even with the statistical need, we have to ask whether the information is accurately reflecting these patient groups. From the example in Figure 5.3, the information obtained could not be relied upon in terms of its accuracy.

Activity 5.7   *Critical thinking*

Look at the options presented to patients in Figure 5.3. What do you think of these, in terms of assessing patients' ethnic/cultural background? Try to give reasons for your opinions.

An outline answer is given at the end of this chapter.

White British	White Irish ✓	White other	White & Black Caribbean
White & Black African	White & Asian	Other mixed	Indian & Asian/ British Asian
Asian & British Asian/Pakistani	Asian & British Asian/ Bangladeshi	Other Asian	Black Caribbean & Black British
Black African & Black British	Other Black	Chinese	Any other group

Figure 5.3: Who are you?

In general, the idea of understanding ethnic/cultural backgrounds helps to inform the statistics held by the Office for National Statistics, which is also responsible for the country's census, the latest being in 2011. In health care, assessing for ethnic/cultural breakdown helps us to understand disease patterns among different groups of the population. Different ethnic groups are prone to certain illnesses. For example, black African men over 50 years of age are more likely to develop prostate cancer (www.prostatecanceruk.org) when compared to other ethnic groups, and this is important in planning appropriate interventions.

For health care policy makers, commissioners and service providers, obtaining ethnic/cultural information helps to create a picture of which groups of the population access their services, and tailor the care to their cultural needs. It is clear that there are good intentions for assessing ethnic backgrounds of patients, but, as already discussed above, we have to be mindful that such information may at some point be inaccurate because of the cultural modifications as time goes on.

What can be done?

It is not easy to recommend ideas that will meet every patient's need. However, if we start by talking openly about death and dying (Nyatanga 2013), we may end up not focusing too much on cultural differences, but on the patient as a person we need to care for. I have argued elsewhere that talking openly about death and dying is seen as one major step towards achieving a unique death, as desired by the dying patient (Department of Health 2008; Nyatanga 2013). By focusing on the patient as a person and not a cultural being, we recognise and respect the uniqueness of all patients, and thereby understand their needs and aspirations for the remaining time of their life.

It is also important to consider the idea of 'meet me halfway', which requires both patients and health care professionals to make an effort to get to know each other. 'Meet me halfway' is a simple but effective concept that tries to educate people on values and beliefs that guide our different lives. To be successful, the concept requires closer integration by minority ethnic communities into wider society, learning the language and appreciating the social etiquette inherent in that society. Equally, the major culture (society) needs to be sensitive to the needs of minority groups. What tends to happen is that we can turn cultural differences into societal strength as we begin to work closely together.

It is therefore important that introspection takes place in an honest way so that we can understand ourselves in the face of difference.

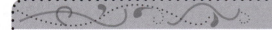 Chapter summary

This chapter has discussed a number of issues to do with culture and the need for cultural competence, which is important for student nurses. We discussed the term culture, which is often used loosely and therefore lacks a clear definition. The term culture is used so broadly that it covers all aspects of our life. For example, socially, culture may refer to music trends, dance types, food and drink, clothes, sex, sports and other hobbies. In health care, culture may refer to a way of caring in a particular hospital or ward/unit or out in the community. As a society, we may use the term culture to refer to race, nationality, ethnicity, rituals, heritage and traditions. It is clear from the above that culture refers to different things about

continued ...

people's characteristics – behaviour, preferences or rituals. The culture we are most concerned with is that which guides how different patients and family pursue their values and belief systems, leading to how they prefer to be cared for and die.

We discussed the impact of acculturation on individual patients and also on us as health care professionals. This led us into the idea of multicultural society and how health care professionals can be competent when caring in such an environment. This led to the discussion about the need for cultural competence and the challenges inherent in this idea.

Whilst cultural competence is a noble idea, the cultural world around it is changing and therefore we need to start planning for care that reflects the future. This is an important realisation and we should try and look at cultural care in a different way. As part of that implementation plan, it is important that we learn from the experiences of palliative care providers already working closely with different cultural communities. The efforts of numerous hospices, for example, attempt to provide care which is culturally sensitive, and by implication that which is accessible and acceptable to culturally diverse populations. The cornerstone of hospice work centres around engaging with local ethnic communities, working in partnership, as a means of achieving community outreach and dialogue – a lesson that can be useful in other settings.

A commitment to education and training now is worthwhile as it is a valid investment that guarantees improved quality of care, which is also culturally sensitive at the end of life.

Activities: brief outline answers

Activity 5.4: Critical thinking

Cultural competence can be summarised in two broad ways – ability and knowledge – and explained thus:

- ability to interact effectively with and care for people of different cultures from your own;
- have knowledge-based skills to provide effective clinical care to patients from different ethnic or racial groups.

Activity 5.6: Critical thinking

Competence is an ongoing quality and therefore the challenge is:

- How do we know that someone is competent?
- How do we assess it, and how often? For example, someone can be competent today but may not be next week.
- There is no accepted standard measure for such competence.
- Another challenge is that there may be people who are just competent and others who may extremely competent, so what would be an acceptable level of competence?
- To be culturally competent would not be enough in a multicultural society like the UK, as you need to be multiculturally competent as well.

- Another challenge is to do with language and whether we will be able to understand and speak all the different languages our patients speak.
- How do we ensure there is cultural desire in all health care professionals?

Activity 5.7: Critical thinking

- It is not clear what the different categories are trying to achieve, as these options are not the same (uniform).
- Some options, like white or black, focus on skin colour, whereas options like white and Asian refer to a product of marriage between the two groups.
- The other options focus on country of birth/origin, like: Pakistani, Indian, British and Bangladeshi, while others refer to continents where people come from, like Asian, African.
- It is important to point out that the patient may have had his/her values influenced by different backgrounds, and therefore the range of options in this activity may not accurately capture the patient's cultural background.
- Consequently, the care offered and services provided may be based on inaccurate information. This may explain why most people from the BME community still do not access the palliative care services that are on offer in the UK.
- One final point to make is the 'Other' option, as it is hard to make sense of who this group is and their values.

Further reading

Gilbert, P. (2013) (ed.) *Spirituality and End of Life Care.* Hove: Pavillion Publishing.

Although the title is Spirituality, this book discusses important aspects of end of life care. For example, there are chapters on a good death as well as on dignity in end of life care. You may find parts 1–5 most relevant as you start your new career in nursing and palliative care.

Oliviere, D., Munroe, B. and Payne, S. (2011) *Death, Dying, and Social Differences,* 2nd edn. Oxford: Oxford University Press.

This book discusses key aspects of cultural, ethnic and social differences. It is relevant to palliative care, and is written by experts in the field. It is easy to read and informative.

Useful websites

www.ons.gov.uk/ons/rel/census/2011-census/population-and-household-estimates-for-the-united-kingdom/stb-2011-census--population-estimates-for-the-united-kingdom.html

This website gives population estimates for the UK.

www.statistics.gov.uk

This website provides a gateway to national statistics of the UK's population, including culture, equality and diversity, which are areas of interest in relation to this chapter.

www.prostatecanceruk.org

This website is owned by Prostate Cancer UK, and aims to raise awareness about prostate cancer. It encourages men, with the support of their families, to be tested early for the disease. It also gives information on developments and recommended treatments.

Chapter 6
Ethical issues in palliative and end of life care

Sherri Ogston-Tuck

NMC Standards for Pre-registration Nursing Education

This chapter will address the following competencies:

Domain 1: Professional values

1. All nurses must practise with confidence according to *The Code: Standards of Conduct, Performance and Ethics for Nurses and Midwives* (NMC 2008), and within other recognised ethical and legal frameworks. They must be able to recognise and address ethical challenges relating to people's choices and decision making about their care, and act within the law to help them and their families and carers find acceptable solutions.

Domain 2: Communication and interpersonal skills

2. All nurses must use a ranges of communication skills and technologies to support person-centred care and enhance quality and safety. They must ensure people receive all the information they need in a language and manner that allows them to make informed choices and share decision making. They must recognise when language interpretation or other communication support is needed and know how to obtain it.

Domain 4: Leadership, management and team working

4. All nurses must be self-aware and recognise how their own values, principles and assumptions may affect their practice. They must maintain their own personal and professional development, learning from experience, through supervision, feedback, reflection and evaluation.

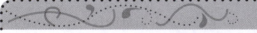

NMC Essential Skills Clusters

This chapter will address the following:

Cluster: Care, compassion and communication

3. People can trust the newly registered graduate nurse to respect them as individuals and strive to help them preserve their dignity at all times.

First progression point

1. Demonstrates respect for diversity and individual preferences, valuing differences, regardless of personal view.

Entry to the register

6. Acts autonomously to challenge situations or others when someone's dignity may be compromised.

4. People can trust a newly qualified graduate nurse to engage with them and their family or carers within their cultural environments in an acceptable and anti-discriminatory manner free from harassment and exploitation.

First progression point

3. Adopts a principled approach to care underpinned by *The Code* (NMC 2008).

Entry to the register

5. Is acceptant of differing cultural traditions, beliefs, UK legal frameworks and professional ethics when planning care with people and their families and carers.

Chapter aims

After reading this chapter you will be able to:

- understand the theories and principles of medical and health care ethics;
- consider your role in recognising ethical and legal challenges relating to palliative and end of life care;
- reflect on your own values and thoughts about people's choices and decision making about their care at end of life;
- explore the role of the nurse in relation to ethical issues in palliative care.

Introduction

Maria wanted to be a nurse for as long as she could remember . . . she believed that she would be a good nurse. But five years on since her qualification, Maria has started to question this. Am I a good nurse? I don't feel like I am making a difference . . .

Questioning whether someone is a good nurse may be helpful in understanding what ethics means in nursing practice. Ethics in itself is about 'what is good', in contrast to 'what is right'. However it is not as simple as debating the nature of good nursing – this would not make Maria a 'good' nurse. Understanding how people become good nurses will help to underpin our understanding of ethics in nursing, and in health care practice.

Ethics is not something separate from patient care that you only think about occasionally (Hawley 2007). The very nature of ethics requires you to reflect on your actions, to consider reasons for those actions and outcomes. This requires consideration of anticipated outcomes, and more importantly, the decisions made and consequences of your actions. Serious engagement in ethics highlights some of the tensions between nursing as an ethical role and as a professional, legal or institutional role (Tingle and Cribb 2007). Health care is becoming increasingly more technically advanced. New medicines, treatment options and surgical procedures are available where they were not before. Difficult decisions are being made where once there would have been no decision to make, because the option simply was not there. People are undergoing more radical treatment that extends the quantity of their life, but not necessarily its quality. For patients with a terminal diagnosis, it is important that they are involved in the decision-making process and have the ability to steer the direction of their treatment. Strategies like advance care planning allow patients to participate in this process actively and decide what treatment they may or may not wish to have in the future. These changes have increased and heightened the importance of nursing ethics that emphasises professional accountability, policy, frameworks and guidelines, and personal responsibility. Ethics asks you to consider what is right and wrong, and challenges you to reflect on your own belief systems. This chapter will support you in your ability to apply an ethical framework to your clinical practice. It will encourage you to consider the ethical issues that are evident in palliative and end of life care.

What is ethics?

Your professional role demands that you consider the ethical implications of decisions made in your day-to-day practice. Ethics in clinical practice can be regarded as quality care (Bishop and Scudder 2001), where the ethical ideal of caring requires you to be culturally sensitive and competent (Hawley 2007). Beliefs are certain principles which we argue should be followed by other people, and which we use as a standard for our own personal behaviour. These everyday ethical reflections amid judgements are important.

In nursing and health care practice ethics is rarely approached as a separate entity from both legal and professional dimensions. Together, they help you to question what is good (ethical dimension) and what is right (legal dimension) and in making decisions and taking action (professional dimension) for patients in your care. It is from the outcome of these, and indeed the role of the nurse, that ethics may be understood more clearly. As a nurse, your goal is to promote health and to prevent harm, and to some extent perhaps this is what Maria is questioning when she asks herself whether she is a good nurse.

The values that shape nursing practice reflect the nature of the nurse–patient relationship and elicit ideas such as empowerment, partnership and advocacy. Nursing ethics involves making decisions and value judgements about nursing care and 'what is good nursing'.

At the centre of this is patient care, but what are the aims of care? What you value in nursing care reflects your professional role to deliver good care, and the decisions you make to provide safe and effective care and promote health and well-being. The values built into this and your delivery of care underpins ethics, and the principles of ethics. This is about values, choice and judgements. Many of the key ethical issues nurses face stem from what nurses perceive their role to be – that of a good nurse – and of the care they give: good care.

The term ethics is used broadly in the context of our values and morals: what we perceive to be good or bad, right or wrong. It also encompasses professionalism – 'professional ethics'. According to Beauchamp and Childress (2009) ethics is a generic term covering several different ways of examining and understanding the 'moral life'. Seeking to 'act ethically' or to 'be ethical' requires first recognising that a moral situation exists. A moral situation forces you to think about what you would want for yourself, how you would want to be treated, and what you value as an individual, and then to extend this to your patients. An ethical issue can arise from any of the following:

- when you have to judge what is right or wrong;
- choosing between options;
- deciding whether to do something or do nothing;
- asking yourself: should I or shouldn't I?;
- weighing up the potential impact of your decisions or actions;
- a dilemma – making a difficult choice.

Your understanding of the concepts of right and wrong is inherent, where you consciously have a grasp of the core dimensions of morality: not to lie; not to steal; to respect others; not to kill or cause harm to innocent persons. Therefore 'common morality' is a concept shared by all people, who are committed to morality. In ethics, this gives rise to rules of obligations, which are moral characteristics or virtues.

Virtues in ethics are questions about your character – qualities of character; admirable or desirable dispositions. This is important in nursing ethics, and helps to answer what it is that makes you a 'good nurse'.

Activity 6.1   *Critical thinking*

Think for a moment about how you would describe yourself.

What morals or virtues do you hold?

Of the list of virtues below, choose those that you feel are necessary for nursing:

Honesty	Integrity	Truthfulness	Loyalty	Patience	Humility
Courage	Resilience				

Would you add anything to this list?

Brief answers to all activities are given at the end of the chapter.

In completing Activity 6.1 it is likely that the words you used to describe yourself were also reflected in the morals/virtues you felt were necessary for nursing. This allows you to see that the morals you hold as a person have the potential to influence how you are as a nurse, highlighting the potential for dilemmas to occur.

What is an ethical dilemma?

Ethical issues in health care are defined as those phenomena or behaviours that have the potential to become a problem (Hawley 2007). Ethical problems are those incidents or situations that have arisen from a moral or ethical issue and which are vitally important in the life of the patient. The following are examples of questions that raise intrinsic philosophical matters to do with the nature and value of life:

- Is it right that someone should be left to die in pain, without choice, because it is a fundamental human right to life?
- Is it wrong to end life, where there is suffering and futility of life?

In health care, ethics refers to a wide range of practice situations. There are few decisions, actions or omissions that do not have an ethical dimension (Beauchamp and Childress 2009). It is impossible to treat these issues seriously without some consideration of moral and ethical questioning. Doing this generates awareness of your own limitations. However, being 'philosophically skilled' does not necessarily mean being a good person but it does mean taking an interest in your character as well as your actions (Tingle and Cribb 2007).

It is possible – sometimes all too easy – not to do what you regard as the right thing. Ethics in health care is about doing the right thing in a certain situation and being a certain kind of person in that situation (Gallagher and Hodge 2012). There are some ethical 'rules' that can be applied to your practice. These underpin your professional role, morals and conscience, and virtues:

- veracity – truth telling, informed consent, respect for autonomy;
- privacy – a person's right to remain private, not to disclose information;
- confidentiality – only sharing private information on a 'need to know' basis;
- fidelity – loyalty, maintaining the duty to care for all, no matter who they are or what they may have done.

Activity 6.2   *Reflection*

Of the list of ethical rules above, which of these do you possess as a virtue?

An outline answer is given at the end of this chapter.

You may have found that some of the ethical rules you said you possess in Activity 6.2 mirror those qualities that you listed in Activity 6.1. These underlying virtues and rules underpin your response to specific situations. To support you in your decision making we will now discuss some of the theories used in ethics.

Theories in ethics

Before considering theories of ethics and their differences there are some other aspects of ethics that need to be considered. Ethics has to do with 'how people act' and 'how people behave' and as a starting point can be broadly separated into *consequentialism*, taking the consequences of your actions into consideration, and *deontology*, basing your actions on a set of principles or duties.

Normative ethics is concerned with what people 'should or ought to do' and how they should live. For you as a nurse aiming to promote health and prevent harm, this can present a dilemma. Non-normative ethics (or *descriptive ethics*) seeks to establish the facts of a situation, not what ought to be done. Normative ethics is concerned with what people 'should or ought to do' and how they should live. For you as a nurse aiming to promote health and prevent harm, this can present a dilemma. It is a form of inquiry to answer the question of moral norms (also called practical or applied ethics) whereas in non-normative ethics (also called descriptive or metaethics) this aims to investigate the facts of moral conduct of how people reason or act (Beauchamp and Childress 2009). For example, determining which moral norms and attitudes are expressed in professional practice. In nursing this would be derived from your professional code of conduct or determined from the organisational mission statement or policy. Non-normative ethics seeks to establish the facts of a situation, not what ought to be done. The scenario below illustrates how both normative and non-normative ethics are evident in your clinical practice.

Scenario

Staff nurse Maria is caring for an elderly man who is recovering from hip surgery. William is 82, has been a widower for six years and lives alone with his dog, Charlie. He has had Charlie for nine years. One day William fell on the pavement whilst walking Charlie. William walks Charlie three times a day; during these walks William often has a cigarette. While in hospital William misses this routine and to some extent his ritual; he often goes outside to have a cigarette. Maria finds it difficult to help William. She knows that smoking will not be good for his wound healing and overall health. William does not see how this is going to impair his health. Up until his fall, he had never been into hospital.

In this situation normative ethics is evident in that William does not feel that his routine is causing him ill health; he does not feel the need to change his lifestyle. Maria is approaching this from a non-normative ethics perspective. She knows what the facts of the situation are. Smoking impairs wound healing, therefore to improve his health William should not smoke.

Empirical ethics can be used to support your nursing practice. Generally, empirical ethics involves data collection from questions, focus groups or observations about people and their actions, thoughts, feelings and behaviours. Empirical ethics informs your practice and, in many ways, highlights the importance and relevance of research and evidence-based practice. To explore this theory let us develop the scenario with Maria and William further.

Activity 6.3   *Critical thinking*

A recent survey on patients recovering from hip and knee surgery found that health promotion in the form of diet, exercise and change of lifestyle habits was key to their recovery
time and decreased length of stay in hospital.

How does this help Maria and her dilemma in caring for William?

An outline answer is given at the end of this chapter.

Utilitarianism

Utilitarianism is often referred to as a consequentialist-based theory. This is because it involves
weighing up the consequences of an action. It holds that actions are right or wrong according
to the balance of their good or bad consequences. This theory concentrates on the value of
well-being or intrinsic good, such as happiness and pleasure, freedom and health, welfare and
preference satisfaction. This can be illustrated in the scenario on page 109. It could be considered that William's desire to smoke provides him with pleasure and happiness that he feels
outweigh the bad consequences of smoking. For William, smoking might support him to manage his stress about being in hospital and the fact that he is separated from Charlie. Maria's
dilemma is recognising this and trying to balance the good and bad consequences of William's
actions each time he leaves the ward and goes outside for a cigarette. Her duty of care is not
to harm William and it would be unlawful for Maria physically to stop William from going
outside. However she is obligated to provide him with sufficient information so that he is aware
of the risks and understands these when making autonomous decisions for himself. It would
be unethical for Maria not to consider both sides of this dilemma, but she cannot stop William
from exercising his own free will and choice. The obligation in this scenario is to respect
William and his decisions; this is the moral dilemma Maria faces. With utilitarianism it is the
end or consequences that are important and dictate whether the action is ethical. It is measured in a positive or negative relation to good or happiness and pain or unhappiness (time is
immaterial).

Kantianism

Kantianism, or deontological theory, is modelled on 'moral worth' and 'moral acceptability'. It
can be described as duty-based or an obligation. In health care this obligation would include
respect for individuals. In the scenario above, you can see how Maria has an ethical dilemma, in
trying to help William recover and to promote his health. Her duty of care is not to harm William
but, by letting him leave the ward to smoke, this could lead to harm. Kant's theory of duty
involves holding some features or actions as good in themselves, regardless of their consequences.
One of Kant's most important claims is that the moral worth of an individual's action depends
exclusively on the moral acceptability of the rule (or 'maxim'). The rule provides a moral reason
that justifies the action (Beauchamp and Childress 2009).

Activity 6.4   *Critical thinking*

Using the information in the scenario, can you identify the moral reasoning that justifies Maria's actions?

An outline answer is given at the end of this chapter.

Rights theory or 'liberal individualism'

This is not a new development in moral and political theory (Beauchamp and Childress 2009). It employs the language of rights – civil, political and legal rights – in protecting individuals. Rights-based ethical theory makes claims that are justified; this is a basis for both international and national frameworks in ethical practice. It offers some positive rights – this requires something of others – and some negative rights – this requires that people are left alone without interference. However, rights are not absolute, even the right to life (as evidenced by common moral judgements such as killing in war). Therefore it is necessary to balance claims and distinguish between a violation of a right (an unjustified action against a right) and an infringement of a right (a justified action overriding a right) (Nielson (1993), cited in Beauchamp and Childress (2009)). Returning to the scenario on page 109, stopping William from smoking may be a violation of his right to make choices, whether good or bad, for himself. But if the risk is great and goes against Maria's obligation to prevent harm, this infringement may be justified.

Communitarianism

This theory holds communal values such as the common good, social goals, traditional practices and cooperative virtues, all of which are fundamental in ethics. Virtues-based ethics offers the theoretical approach that focuses on character and ethical qualities or those dispositions of health care professionals.

Activity 6.5   *Critical thinking*

Which virtues does Maria need to demonstrate when caring for William?

An outline answer is given at the end of this chapter.

You may have identified in Activity 6.5 that Maria must demonstrate respect and compassion for William. These virtues reflect the professional values of nurses as described in *The Code* (NMC 2008). As you can see, many theories in ethics are moral-like, where one has to think through the ethical implications of one's decisions and actions. As a result of these different ways of thinking and doing, conflict exists. To support you in working your way through these conflicts you could use an ethical framework.

Ethical frameworks

Beauchamp and Childress's (2009) principles of biomedical ethics (or the principalist approach) address four key moral principles: autonomy, beneficence, non-maleficence and justice. It provides a broad framework that can be used for ethical deliberation and discussion, most notably in health care practice. The principles consider deciding how to act (Tingle and Cribb 2007), where health care professionals ought to respect autonomy and avoid harm, where possible benefit the patient and consider (fairly) the interests of all those affected. Although this framework has been highly criticised as being too simplistic and too mechanical, it offers a critical and thoughtful approach to support you in your ethical decision making. It is important to note, however, that *not all* ethical thinking can be reduced to a few key words or that four principles will provide a quick and easy method for you to use when approaching ethical dilemmas. Rather, the principalist approach provides a reminder of key dimensions of ethical thinking (Tingle and Cribb 2007).

Autonomy

The principle of autonomy recognises the rights of individuals to self-determination. It acknowledges individuals' rights to hold views, make choices and take actions based on their personal values and beliefs (Beauchamp and Childress 2009). Autonomy is an important social value in terms of what is important to the patient, rather than to you as a nurse and to other health care professionals. It is also an indicator of what health means to a patient. Individuals can experience loss of autonomy if they are unwell and no longer able to participate in their life in the way they once did. Overall, having autonomy can be a general indicator of health. For you, as a nurse, respecting autonomy involves supporting rules and obligations to tell the truth, respect for privacy and maintaining confidentiality (Beauchamp and Childress 2009). Key components of this principle require you to respect patients' rights to make their own decisions, to teach people to be able to make their own choices and to support this without force or coercion. An important outcome of this principle is informed consent and it is also the basis for advance care directives.

Activity 6.6   *Critical thinking*

Jenny is 18 and a devout Jehovah's Witness. She has been involved in a car accident. On arrival to the Accident and Emergency department Jenny is haemorrhaging and in need of a blood transfusion. She is conscious and aware of the life-saving treatment proposed, but refuses to have the blood because of her beliefs.

Consider the following questions:

- How will the nurse respect Jenny's autonomy?
- What should she do?

An outline answer is given at the end of this chapter.

In Activity 6.6 you may have identified that the nurse would need to provide Jenny with enough information for her to be able to make an informed decision about her treatment. You may also have to recognise that Jenny may not be fully autonomous and therefore not legally competent to refuse treatment (see Chapter 8 for further information on refusing treatment). An autonomous decision does not have to be the 'correct' decision, otherwise individual needs and values would not be respected. Rather, an autonomous decision is one that is an informed decision.

Non-maleficence

The principle of non-maleficence is embodied by the main consideration to 'do no harm'. You should not cause pain or suffering; should not incapacitate or cause offence; should not deprive people; should not kill.

It is more important not to harm your patients than to do them good. For health care professionals, this influences every intervention, treatment and decision that is made for patients. It is believed that these will do good; however, first you need to consider whether they do no, or acceptable, levels of harm. Non-maleficence underpins evidence-based practice (as does the principle of beneficence – doing good). This relates to issues of consent, and understanding whether treatment is likely to be harmful. The patient should understand the risks and benefits, and that the likely benefits outweigh the likely risks. Unfortunately this principle is not absolute, and must also be balanced against the principle of beneficence.

Activity 6.7   *Critical thinking*

Ms Roberts is 35 and lives with her 15-year-old daughter; she has chronic kidney disease and is in need of dialysis. Ms Roberts is competent to make decisions about her treatment; she is refusing treatment because she is scared of the treatment, which she believes is invasive. She has been counselled about the nature of the treatment and that there are no alternatives that would be of practical benefit. She understands that if she refuses dialysis she will die. The nurse feels very strongly that Ms Roberts should receive dialysis but despite numerous attempts to persuade her, Ms Roberts refuses.

To help you understand this principle, ask yourself the following – remember this principle requires you to do no harm to your patient:

- Would the patient be harmed by the treatment, i.e. by forcibly restraining the patient to carry out the procedure? How will Ms Roberts be affected if she is not treated now?
- Would it be impractical to carry it out if Ms Roberts does not comply? And if so, which course of action would result in the greatest harm?
- How successful is the treatment and are there any alternatives?

An outline answer is given at the end of this chapter.

Activity 6.7 highlights the dilemmas faced by both patients and health care professionals. In this scenario they both know that the long-term outcome of not having dialysis will be death. In addition it could be argued that it is selfish or unfair of Ms Roberts to allow her 15-year-old daughter to watch as her health deteriorates.

Beneficence

The principle of beneficence is one of the core values of health care ethics and is considered in relation to non-maleficence and preventing harm where you 'ought to do good'. It requires weighing up what it means to do good as opposed to what will bring about harm or wrong (Gallagher and Hodge 2012). The term beneficence refers to actions that promote the well-being of others, such as creating a safe and supportive environment and helping people in crisis. Our actions must aim to 'benefit' people – their health, welfare, comfort and well-being, improving a person's potential and quality of life.

Importantly, 'benefit' should be defined by the individuals themselves. It is not what you think that is important. In the medical context, this means taking actions that serve the best interests of patients. This means acting on behalf of vulnerable people, to protect their rights and prevent them from harm. However, uncertainty surrounds the precise definition of which practices do in fact help patients. This is true of end of life care and quality of life issues.

Activity 6.8   *Critical thinking*

Simon is 56, in a hospice, and dying of terminal cancer. Morphine is prescribed to help alleviate his pain and keep him comfortable. However, at the same time, the side-effects of the potent opioid analgesic are causing Simon to feel nauseated, he is often vomiting and he is very drowsy. His family are concerned that, although his pain is gone, he is still suffering. Simon refuses to eat and is refusing any further treatment.

To help you understand this principle, ask yourself the following – remember this principle requires you act to benefit the patient. It may also clash with the principle of respect for autonomy when the patient makes a decision that the health care professional does not think will benefit the patient – not in the patient's 'best interests'.

- How can the balance to benefit Simon while minimising the harmful side-effects of treatment be achieved?
- Is there a benefit to having the patient's autonomy overridden?
- Have both the long-term and short-term effects been considered? Without treatment, will Simon suffer more? Would continued treatment hasten his death or prolong his pain and suffering?

An outline answer is given at the end of this chapter.

The scenario in Activity 6.8 poses a difficult dilemma. It would be helpful if you were aware of an advance care directive (see Chapter 8 for further information) that tells you Simon's wishes for his end of life care. It is also important that his family are aware of his wishes, so that Simon's autonomy is respected and decisions are made in his best interests, which may well be to die with dignity, without pain and without suffering. The benefits of acting beneficently would need to be weighed against the benefits of failing to respect Simon's autonomy. From a legal point of view the wishes of competent patients cannot be overridden in their best interests.

Justice

The principle of justice is about you treating people fairly and not favouring some individuals/ groups over others. You should act in a non-discriminatory or non-prejudicial way. It is also about what is fair and just in the distribution of limited health resources, and the decision as to who gets what treatment. Underlying this principle is equality, which is both challenging and often difficult to grasp in practice. It is based on need, effort, contribution and management. Everyone and everything has an equal share and this principle underpins respect for people's rights and respect for the law.

> **Case study**
>
> *It was recommended that Mrs Otley be treated with an anticancer drug called Avastin. The trust refused to fund the treatment on the basis that the use of the drug as part of a 'cocktail' had not been researched. The court held that insufficient weight had been given to the fact that the proposed treatment was the only one available. Mrs Otley was entitled to have the chance of life (R (Otley) v Barking & Dagenham NHS PCT [2007]). In this case, the issue of cost as such is not relevant; rather, of greater importance is the potential benefit for the individual. However, the difficult decision must be made involving the provision of very expensive life-saving/life-prolonging drugs (Gallagher and Hodge 2012).*

What is fair and just is very difficult to determine in this case study, with both cost and the greater good being contributing factors. In some cases the cost of treatment has to be the trade-off, where other treatment options are available and cheaper. This will override what is fair versus what is just. For the trust sufficient evidence to support the treatment options is the deciding factor. Interestingly, the courts have favoured the benefit of treatment as fair and just where the cost was not relevant and may set a precedent for other patients.

You can apply the four principles approach to real-life cases. The process of standing back, drawing on reflection, engaging in discussion and debate will provide you with a practical framework. Although this approach has its limitations (Gallagher and Hodge 2012), it is very helpful in structuring how you think through the ethical problems that underpin your professional actions.

Jean has had a chronic cough for some time and also has a reduced appetite. She has been worried about her cough and thinks it might be cancer. Her daughter, who is 25, and has been worried about her mother, insisted that she saw a doctor. However, Jean did not do this and her breathlessness is now getting worse, resulting in her being taken to Accident and Emergency. At Accident and Emergency Jean says to the nurse, 'Please don't tell my daughter it is cancer! I know it is. Please, I don't want her to know'.

While at Accident and Emergency Jean's condition rapidly deteriorates and she is ventilated to support her airway and breathing. Her daughter is crying and concerned and wants to know what will happen to her mother. Tests reveal that she has advanced lung cancer and that it is inoperable and terminal.

Now answer the following questions:

- Is the patient autonomous?
- What does it mean to respect the patient's autonomy?
- What are the benefits to be gained?
- What harm, if any, might result from the action taken?
- What is the most just response in this situation?

An outline answer is given at the end of this chapter.

High-quality patient care

When caring for patients receiving palliative and end of life care it is important for you to recognise that relatives need to be assured that high-quality care will be delivered and that the wishes of the patient will be respected (Andershed 2006). In 2008 the Department of Health highlighted that, although some patients receive excellent care at the end of life, many do not. Further studies identified that relatives felt supported and experienced peace of mind when they knew that nurses and other health care professionals were acting in their dying loved one's best interest (Oberle and Hughes 2001; Gott et al. 2004). The importance of nurses and other health care professionals developing a trusting relationship with an open, positive attitude has been identified as an important factor in palliative and end of life care. In addition, being sensitive to the needs of relatives for information and education through effective communication has been recognised (Oberle and Hughes 2001; Andershed 2006).

Sarah is 84. She was admitted to hospital five days ago with pneumonia. Her condition is now deteriorating. She is distressed and semiconscious. Her breathing is laboured, even with oxygen being administered. She moans audibly on expiration, suggesting she is in a great deal of pain and discomfort. Her relatives have asked the staff about her breathing and are also worried that she is in pain. The multiprofessional team discuss Sarah's situation and agreement is reached, but not supported by all staff, that Sarah will be prescribed morphine to control the pain. Some staff are concerned this may compromise Sarah's already weak respiratory system. Others feel that, while morphine may cause respiratory depression, the effect of the drug will relax Sarah's respiratory muscles and she will not have to work as hard to breathe and therefore she will have less pain.

Now consider the following questions and apply the ethical principles to your decision making:

- Are staff correct in their assumption that morphine will compromise the already weakened respiratory system? If so, why? If not, why not?
- Do you think this is the right treatment for Sarah? If so, why? If not, why not?
- What information would you provide to Sarah's family and how?

An outline answer is given at the end of this chapter.

There may not be a right or wrong answer for the questions in Activity 6.10. However, one thing is certain: the nurse has an important role in this situation.

The *End of Life Care Strategy* (Department of Health 2008) recommends that the following qualities contribute towards what is a 'good death'. Patients, their relatives and carers are treated as individuals and they are treated with dignity and respect. Patients are without pain and other symptoms, they are in familiar surroundings and they are in the company of close family and/or friends. Nurses and other health care professionals who demonstrate care and support for a patient's relatives increase the possibility that relatives will develop insight into the patient's health situation and participate in the care in a meaningful way. Here you can see how key concepts that characterise the role of the nurse and other health care professionals link to principles in ethics: respect, openness, sincerity, honesty and compassion. How you care for the dying is an indicator of how you care for all sick and vulnerable people. It is a measure of society as a whole and it is a litmus test for health and social care services (Department of Health 2008).

Quality care in the terminal stages of life

For over ten years now the Liverpool Care Pathway for the Dying Patient (LCP) has been used to support care in the terminal (the last one to two) days of life. The LCP was designed to allow people with a terminal illness to die with dignity, with the care provided being directed at comfort and maintaining the patient's dignity, as well as providing information and support for families. The LCP provided alerts, guidance and a structured single record for nurses, other health care professionals and multidisciplinary teams that are inexpert in palliative care.

However, one of the central issues that caused difficulty in the use of the LCP stemmed from misunderstanding and uncertainty over whether deciding to implement the LCP was a treatment decision that required the patient's consent or, if the patient lacked capacity, required the decision to be taken in the patient's best interests. In some cases, relatives and carers incorrectly considered that they were entitled to decide which treatment their relatives receive. In other cases clinicians failed to seek consent from a patient, or to consult with the relatives and carers in a 'best interests' assessment, when treatment was being changed.

This led to an independent review of the LCP taking place in 2013. The findings were published in the document *More Care, Less Pathway: A Review of the Liverpool Care Pathway* (Independent Review of the Liverpool Care Pathway 2013). As a result it is planned that by the end of 2014 the LCP will be phased out and instead patients will be provided with an 'end of life care plan'. This reminds us that all people approaching the end of life should have their needs assessed, their wishes respected and their preferences discussed, hence the need to plan care.

Patients' plan of care should reflect their choices and include an agreed set of actions identifying how these will be met. This might include an indication of their general wishes and preferences about how they are cared for in the future and where they would wish to die. Is an advance care directive in place for those who may lack capacity to make such decisions in the future? If so, then do the relevant people know about this? What is included and where can it be accessed? All these aspects should be incorporated into a patient's end of life care plan. Caring for those requiring palliative and end of life care is one of the most important and rewarding areas of care – it is a privilege. It can be considered challenging and emotionally demanding, yet with the requisite knowledge, skills and attitudes, it can also be immensely satisfying (Department of Health 2008).

Conclusion

Professional behaviour and standards of care underpin your role as a nurse and the care you deliver professionally, legally and morally. Importantly, reflecting on your own personal beliefs and values has an impact on your clinical and ethical decision making. This is of particular relevance in everyday practice, but even more significant in end of life care, where decision making is not as simple or straightforward. The use of ethical principles and frameworks can help to guide your decision making, and remind you where, and how, your own values and virtues can influence decisions made, hopefully for the better. However, achieving individual ethical integrity in life is difficult (Tschudin 2003, cited in Benjamin and Curtis 2010). In clinical practice, this needs to be inclusive of the multidisciplinary team, open communication and planning individual patient care. When you are faced with ethical dilemmas, adopting an ethical framework and reflective approach emphasises the importance of patient autonomy and choice in end of life care. Underpinning your ethical practice is the awareness of both your professional and legal obligations, to do good and not harm. The decisions you make should, and will, reflect your morals and values, because as nurses, as human beings, these are intrinsic to not only how you care, but also why you care.

Activities: brief outline answers

Activity 6.1: Critical thinking

You can describe yourself both as a person and as a nurse. Your morals and virtues are those characterisitics that are unique to you; they are also those attributes that you possess in your professional role as a nurse. The virtues necessary for a nurse would include all of these: honesty, integrity, truthfulness, loyalty, patience, humility, courage and resilience. In addition you should be: compassionate, caring, competent, skilled, knowledgeable, kind, empathetic, insightful, open and honest, lawful, considerate, non-discriminatory, respectful, supportive, attentive, aware, facilitative, cooperative and impartial. These attributes and list of virtues reflect the NMC Code (2008).

Activity 6.2: Reflection

Veracity, privacy, confidentiality and fidelity are all essential virtues for a nurse to possess. They reflect those attributes that are essential for nursing and the standards of care and professional behaviour and attitude recommended by the NMC (2008).

Activity 6.3: Critical thinking

Maria can use this empirical data as evidence to inform the information she shares with William to help in his recovery. This reflects the importance of how evidence is used in your practice. In this situation it can offload the judgement William may feel Maria is making, with the evidence or statistics being presented in a way that William can choose to see and use to his advantage, helping to sway his own decision making and autonomy.

Activity 6.4: Critical thinking

For Maria the obligation here is to respect the individual: this is the moral dilemma she faces. Although Maria has a professional duty and obligation to prevent harm, the infringement here may not be justified; William is able to make decisions for himself. Whether you agree or not, Maria would need to be supported by her team and colleagues, and she would need to ensure that she has documented the discussion with William and the decision he has made. In some instances, where patients choose to leave the safety of the ward and go outside, this fundamental right and freedom is upheld but patients are also asked to sign a waiver to this effect. This places the accountability and responsibility on the patient and not the nursing staff.

Activity 6.5: Critical thinking

Maria has demonstrated many of the virtues listed. She is respectful and non-judgemental, and she is honest and acts with compassion and integrity. She also draws on her knowledge and skill and works collaboratively with her team and William.

Activity 6.6: Critical thinking

The nurse has to firstly understand and accept that Jenny is able to make decisions for herself, legally. Jenny's autonomy must be respected. A non-judgemental and empathetic approach is needed whilst also ensuring that Jenny has all of the relevant information to make her decisions. Jenny has the capacity to do this, and even if, in this case, the nurse feels this is an unwise decision, it is Jenny's to make. If Jenny's capacity is in question it is not the nurse alone who would seek to challenge or determine this (see Chapter 8). Jenny needs to understand the risks and benefits of having (and not having) the blood transfusion. An informed decision to refuse treatment must be clearly documented and communicated with the health care team and any alternative treatment equally discussed with Jenny. The nurse cannot give the treatment if Jenny refuses. The nurse and any members of the health care team must also respect Jenny's decision.

Activity 6.7: Critical thinking

Forcing treatment would be conceived as harmful and forcibly restraining Ms Roberts would be unlawful. This would have an impact on trust between Ms Roberts and the nurse, and could indeed cause further harm. Any alternative treatments or therapies must be shared with Ms Roberts, and this information needs to be openly discussed with her. There may well be some success in alternative treatments or this could be a source of greater pain and discomfort. However, the nurse has an obligation to ensure both the risks and benefits of any alternatives, and specialist expertise consultation, are provided to ensure that Ms Roberts's decision is informed. Respecting the patient's wishes in this instance is difficult but necessary. Ms Roberts's autonomy must be respected.

Activity 6.8: Critical thinking

To act in a way that benefits Simon, it is necessary to firstly respect his autonomy and his wishes. Striking a balance between benefit and harm is not easy, and this is where the clash in respecting Simon's choice for himself is the challenge. It is necessary to keep Simon comfortable and painfree; it is also important to manage the side-effects of the pain relief in his best interests. One could argue there is no benefit to overriding Simon's autonomy and to continue treatment. In the short term, he is *less likely* to suffer, but without adequate pain relief, more suffering is likely.

Activity 6.9: Critical thinking

Patient autonomy is about what is important to the patient so in this case it is necessary to understand what the symptoms, and indeed illness, mean for Jean. Whilst Jean is sedated and ventilated the nurse caring for Jean must respect her autonomy and support her decision for her daughter not to be told her diagnosis. Even if there is an underlying obligation to tell Jean's daughter, this truth would not be respectful of Jean's wishes or for her privacy and confidentiality. Jean has the right to make her own decisions and own choices here, however difficult these might be for the nurse. At the moment the health care professionals have a duty of care to Jean, to respect her wishes and to keep her daughter informed of the treatment and care. Respecting Jean's autonomy and making decisions that are in her best interests necessitate a balance, weighing up whether telling the daughter of her terminal prognosis and diagnosis is going to benefit Jean or cause her further harm. The benefit of telling her daughter may cause greater harm and fracture the nurse–patient relationship. Here, the most just response may be in arguing it is in the patient's best interests for her daughter to know that she may not recover, or may not live.

Activity 6.10: Evidence-based practice

This scenario highlights some of the ethical dilemmas present. Staff may have differing views; however, what is important is that when discussing Sarah's treatment with her family and relatives the information they provide is consistent. This will reduce the family's anxiety and promote clear communication. In addition the nurse needs to ensure that Sarah's relatives are well informed and feel that they are involved in her care and treatment in a meaningful way. This will require the nurse, and other health care professionals, to demonstrate feelings of mutual trust and confidence between the patient and family.

Further reading

Casarett, D. (2005) Ethical considerations in end-of-life care and research. *Journal of Palliative Medicine*, 8 (S1): S148–S161.

This article discusses six ethical aspects of end of life care that clinicians and researchers should take into consideration when conducting palliative care research.

Fry, S.T. and Johnstone, M.J. (2002) *Ethics in Nursing Practice: A Guide to Ethical Decision Making*. London: Blackwell.

This book will provide you with an in-depth understanding of the ethical, legal and professional issues that are key in supporting you to maintain professional standards.

Tschudin, V. (ed.) (2003) *Approaches to Ethics: Nursing Beyond Boundaries*, 3rd edn. Edinburgh: Butterworth Heinemann.

This text is a collection of contributions, from internationally recognised authors, on different approaches to ethics. These are written about and applied to nursing contexts.

Wheat, K. (2009) Applying ethical principles in healthcare practice. *British Journal of Nursing*, 18 (17): 1062–1063.

This article outlines general ethical principles that can be applied to all health care contexts.

Useful websites

www.corec.org.uk

The Central Office for Research Ethics website contains useful information for health care professionals.

www.nmc-uk.org

This is the website for the Nursing and Midwifery Council. It contains relevant information about professional standards and guidance for practice.

www.rcn.org.uk

This is the website for the RCN, the largest professional union for nursing in the UK. Their website provides information on professional development and support.

www.scie.org.uk/research/ethics-committee

This website provides you with information about the Social Care Research Ethics Committee. It includes information about the research carried out and how to apply for research ethics review.

Chapter 7
Palliative and end of life care in a critical care setting

Hazel Luckhurst

NMC Standards for Pre-registration Nursing Education

This chapter will address the following competencies:

Domain 1: Professional values

1. All nurses must practise with confidence according to *The Code: Standards of Conduct, Performance and Ethics for Nurses and Midwives* (NMC 2008), and within other recognised ethical and legal frameworks. They must be able to recognise and address ethical challenges relating to people's choices and decision making about their care, and act within the law to help them and their families and carers find acceptable solutions.

Domain 2: Communication and interpersonal skills

3. All nurses must use the full range of communication methods, including verbal, non-verbal and written, to acquire, interpret and record their knowledge and understanding of people's needs. They must be aware of their own values and beliefs and the impact this may have on their communication with others. They must take account of the many different ways in which people communicate and how these may be influenced by ill health, disability and other factors, and be able to recognise and respond effectively when a person finds it hard to communicate.

Domain 3: Nursing practice and decision making

4. All nurses must ascertain and respond to the physical, social and psychological needs of people, groups and communities. They must then plan, deliver and evaluate safe, competent, person-centred care in partnership with them, paying special attention to changing health needs during different life stages, including progressive illness and death, loss and bereavement.

4.2. Adult nurses must recognise and respond to the changing needs of adults, families and carers during terminal illness. They must be aware of how treatment goals and service users' choices may change at different stages of progressive illness, loss and bereavement.

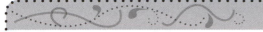

NMC Essential Skills Clusters

This chapter will address the following:

Cluster: Care, compassion and communication

2. People can trust the newly registered graduate nurse to engage in person-centred care empowering people to make choices about how their needs are met when they are unable to meet them for themselves.

Second progression point

6. Provides personalised care, or makes provision for those who are unable to maintain their own activities of living maintaining dignity at all times.

3. People can trust the newly registered graduate nurse to respect them as individuals and strive to help them preserve their dignity at all times.

Entry to the register

4. Acts professionally to ensure that personal judgements, prejudices, values, attitudes and beliefs do not compromise care.

Chapter aims

After reading this chapter you will be able to:

* describe the three suggested phases relating to the management of a patient in critical care;
* identify the challenges of introducing and caring for palliative care patients in a critical care environment;
* reflect on the support required for the patient, family and critical care staff when delivering palliative and end of life care.

Introduction

I will never forget the day I walked into the critical care unit at the hospital to see my son. Simon had been in a road accident and the police brought us to the hospital . . . What a shock. Even though the nurse had explained about Simon's bed area and the tubes before we walked in, I couldn't quite take it all in. As we got near to the bed my husband just collapsed and fell to the floor. We had to give him a few moments on the floor before sitting him up. He had fainted at the sight of Simon in the bed, all swollen, surrounded by machines and equipment.

(A mother's reflection on seeing her son for the first time following a road accident)

You may find a critical care environment alien and frightening; this is also true for families whose loved ones are being cared for in critical care. Simon's mother's words in the quote above recognise this. The focus is on the 'tubes' and 'machines', and the overt impact of this environment on Simon's parents, emphasised by his father's collapse. The very nature of the invasive life-saving treatment in a critical care unit involves monitoring both the patient and equipment at the bedside.

Activity 7.1   *Reflection*

They say, 'A picture paints a thousand words'. Search for images of critical care units on the internet; write down the words that these pictures suggest to you.

Brief answers to all activities are given at the end of the chapter, unless otherwise indicated. This activity is based on your own observations, so there is no outline answer given.

You might have included words like 'technical', 'equipment' or 'frightening' in your reflection in Activity 7.1. In addition to monitoring equipment there is what can be viewed as a seemingly endless number of investigations, such as X-rays and blood tests. All critically ill patients have cables and leads attaching them to equipment that displays their vital signs, for example, heart rhythm and rate. The screens on the equipment display several coloured waveforms and are linked to specific haemodynamics of the patient, e.g. arterial blood pressure, cardiac rhythm and pulse oximetry. Patients receive intravenous infusions and may have several cannulae infusing fluids for hydration and nourishment. Medication will be infused via syringe infusion pumps and bags of intravenous fluids. Additional therapies may also be present at the bedside, such as a renal support machine and a ventilator supporting the patient's respiratory system. Patients in a critical care setting are obviously critically ill, usually with a condition that is reversible, although not always. Sometimes there is the need to introduce the principles for palliative and end of life care (discussed in Chapter 1). Whatever the setting, be it home, hospital ward or critical care, you should look beyond the machines and equipment and afford the *patient, family* and *carers* the best possible care. You should recognise therefore that if you select critical care as a career choice it is important to know that around 20 per cent of patients may not survive their admission (Intensive Care Society 2011). Therefore end of life care is a substantial aspect of day-to-day care for the critical care nurse.

What is a critical care setting?

In the literature and within this chapter we refer to the critical care unit (CCU) and the intensive care unit (ICU). Another term used in the UK is intensive therapy unit (ITU), and these terms are used interchangeably. However, in health care 'critical care' is carried out in many areas within a hospital.

Activity 7.2   *Reflection*

Reflect back on your clinical practice, or personal experience, including images you saw
on the internet, and identify the different types of critical care settings you have heard of.
Once you have done this, spend some time finding out what other critical care units or
intensive care units there are and identify three specialities. Thinking about these specialities, what could the difference be in the types of patients admitted?

An outline answer is given at the end of this chapter.

In your reflection in Activity 7.2 you will have identified a range of settings where critical care is
delivered: ITU settings, theatres or Accident and Emergency departments. Hospital management
teams describe their critical care *service provision* collectively as operating theatres, medical assessment units, high dependency units, admission wards and Accident and Emergency departments.
To put it simply, the critical care unit provides care for seriously and acutely ill (critically ill)
patients who are assessed as having a potentially reversible condition (Adam and Osborne 2005;
Intensive Care Society 2011). It has taken a considerable time to define what happens in intensive
care units around the UK because of the variation in patient criteria, reason for admission and
speciality of some intensive care units. To support ease of understanding across health care settings, a national review by the Department of Health took place in 2000. This review defined four
levels of care throughout the hospital services (Department of Health 2000) (Table 7.1).

Level of care	Place of care
Level 0	Patients whose needs can be met through a normal ward setting
Level 1	Patients at risk of their condition deteriorating, or needing higher levels of care, whose need can be met with advice and support from the critical care team
Level 2	Patients requiring more detailed observation or intervention (single failing organ system) or postoperative care, and higher levels of care
Level 3	Patients requiring advanced respiratory support alone or basic respiratory support together with support of at least two organ systems. This level includes all complex patients requiring support for multiorgan failure

Table 7.1: Defined levels of care (Department of Health 2000)

Patients requiring level 2 and 3 support are usually nursed in an intensive care or critical care
unit. This is because they need potentially life-saving measures requiring staff with specialist skills
and knowledge, in addition to the use of medical technology. As medicine and the speciality of
critical care have advanced, subspecialties of intensive care have evolved. For example, a large
university teaching hospital could have more than one critical care unit. The units may be named

according to their speciality, for example, neurosciences critical care unit, cardiothoracic critical care unit, paediatric and trauma critical care unit.

Within the last decade the profile of end of life care within the critical care environment has been more evident in both UK and international policy and publications (Intensive Care Society 2003; Carlet et al. 2004; Department of Health 2008; Chapman 2009; Stayt 2009; Coombs et al. 2012). The national mortality rate in adult critical care units is approximately 17 per cent (Intensive Care National Audit and Research Centre 2010).

Phases of care in critical care

In terms of planning and implementing individual patient-centred care, nursing patients in critical care is no different from other health care settings. However there are some differences that should be recognised. First, the fundamental aim when a person is admitted to critical care is one of cure and recovery, rather than palliation. Medical technology and interventions actively support and can even replace the function of some organ systems during the severe stages of organ failure. Second, it is often not possible to involve patients in discussions about their care as they are seriously ill, at times unconscious, and may be unable to communicate. Third, the serious illness may have developed rapidly, within minutes or hours, and finally, other services such as a hospice or palliative care teams may have had more time to plan end of life care with the patient and loved ones.

The discussion above and national statistics indicate that mortality in critical care is high. This is why nurses, and other health care staff working in critical care, can be regularly providing end of life care. Using a framework could be helpful for you when considering the process of palliative care in critical care. One framework is described by Coombs et al. (2012), who discuss the following specific trajectory, involving three phases of care in critical care. Each phase will now be described using a supportive case scenario to illustrate what happens to a patient in each phase. Phase 0 is not discussed as it is technically not applicable to the intensive care environment.

Phase 1: hope of recovery

Patients are admitted to the critical care environment because there is *hope of recovery*. This hope of recovery is demonstrated in the example of Aisha below.

Case study

Aisha

Aisha was admitted to the critical care unit. She had developed a respiratory infection 24 hours before admission and her breathing had become increasingly difficult. The paramedic visited her home and immediately transported her to the hospital. She required sedation and respiratory support via a ventilator due to acute respiratory failure and pneumonia. Specific antibiotic therapy was commenced with the hope that Aisha would recover fully.

Looking at this example you may want to argue that this phase does not really require palliative care, as there is still hope for recovery. It is only if Aisha's condition deteriorates that she might move to phase 2, the transition phase. This scenario demonstrates some of the material in Chapter 1, with the idea that palliative care can take place alongside curative care.

Phase 2: the transition stage

This involves recognition that the treatment is not effective in the planned recovery of the patient. Interventions have not resulted in improvement of the patient's condition. There is a process of acknowledgement and a diagnosis that the person is dying. The delivery of care moves from active critical care interventions to palliation and end of life care.

Case study

Steve

Steve was an elective admission to the critical care unit following major surgery to repair an aortic aneurysm. Postoperatively Steve developed sepsis and remained critically ill for five weeks, requiring renal replacement therapy. His respiratory function deteriorated and he required further ventilation. The specific interventions to treat this sepsis and support his failing organ systems were not effective. He continued to be hypotensive despite intravenous infusions of vasoactive drug therapy. Throughout the five weeks of Steve's stay in critical care the staff had developed a rapport with his family. The family had had regular meetings with the staff since admission to discuss Steve's plan of care and recognised that his condition was worse.

When a patient's condition is worsening, health care professionals often review the care and treatment options for that patient. At times some forms of treatment become futile and it takes courage and knowledge to decide against futile treatment. The word futile may not be the easiest to understand, but when used in the caring environment it has a specific meaning. For example, if the multidisciplinary team you work with talks about the current treatment being futile, they mean that the treatment/intervention that the person is receiving is not having a positive effect (*Mosby's Medical Dictionary* 2009). Recognising the futility of treatment is the fundamental aspect of phase 2 in relation to the management of the patient (for further information on non-beneficence, see Chapter 6).

In Steve's case (phase 2) his organs were failing and therefore a decision to withdraw treatment would be made as part of the care plan. There are guidelines (Intensive Care Society 2003) which should be followed when this decision is made. They state that there should be agreement from two senior doctors, with one of the doctors being an intensive care consultant (Cohen et al. 2003). The guidelines also acknowledge that it is 'normal practice' for the opinions of the nursing and other medical team members to be considered. This shared decision-making process is supported by a survey carried out by McAree and Doherty in 2010. When this decision is made, be careful what terminology is used. It is preferable to say 'withdrawing active therapy' rather than 'withdrawal of treatment', because whatever phase patients are in, they are still receiving treatment. Steve, for example, will have the vasoactive drugs and the renal replacement therapy discontinued, but he will continue to receive analgesia, and some support from the ventilator.

> ## Case study
>
> ## Tom
>
> *Tom has been in the ITU, and receiving respiratory support, for the past three weeks. Tom has a long history of chronic obstructive pulmonary disease and has had multiple chest infections over the past six months. He is not responding to the critical care interventions and intravenous antibiotics for this chest infection. He is still not able to breathe without the maximum support of a ventilator. Tom does not appear to be recovering; in fact, he is worse today.*
>
> *The critical care team have recognised that Tom is in phase 2; Tom's care will now move from active critical care interventions to end of life care.*

> ## Activity 7.3   *Critical thinking*
>
> Reflect on Tom's case study.
>
> - What possible feelings might you as the professional experience in this situation?
> - What strategies could you put in place to address these and support yourself?
>
> *An outline answer is given at the end of this chapter.*

Activity 7.3 might have highlighted to you the emotional dilemma that nurses and other professionals working in a critical care setting face. It can be challenging for you as a nurse to make that transition from active treatment to palliation and end of life care. At the same time that the decision is made to withdraw active therapy, the critical care team should discuss the plan for transition to end of life care. As well as including staff, as mentioned above, the views of the relatives are important and will be discussed in detail later in this chapter. Throughout the patient's stay, it is possible and most likely that you will have developed a rapport with the family and close friends of the patient. In critical care the nurse is constantly at the patient's bedside, so is spending much more time with the patient and the family than the medical team and other health care professionals, e.g. physiotherapist, pharmacist. This places you in the ideal position to support the relatives and care for their reactions, needs and feelings (Intensive Care Society 2003; Coombs et al. 2012). In addition this relationship will support you to explain to the relatives and friends about the process that is being undertaken and how decisions will be made. This can be an emotional time for you; it is important, therefore, that all health care professionals and nurses in particular have ways to self-care and debrief during or after each shift.

Phase 3: a controlled death

The term 'controlled death' could conjure up different meanings, including helping someone to die, which would be misconstruing what Coombs et al. (2012) and others had in mind. The phrase 'controlled death' should be viewed as allowing death to take place in a dignified way, through palliation to ease the pain and suffering, recognising the suddenness of the death and the different meaning this has for people. It is necessary to emphasise here that Coombs et al. (2012) expand upon the term as a time of palliation, allowing nature to take its course, saying goodbye and returning the dead person to his or her family.

Case study

Sarah

Sarah arrived in the critical care unit four hours after involvement in a road traffic collision. She was unconscious, and had sustained multiple injuries. At the scene Sarah had required intubation and ventilation to support her breathing. She had undergone emergency abdominal surgery for extensive bleeding due to liver trauma. Assessment by the surgical team concluded that, due to her extensive injuries and damage, no further surgery was possible. While in critical care Sarah had received extensive blood transfusion products but was still unable to maintain an effective circulation. The critical care team discussed the situation with Sarah's family and end of life care commenced. The priority was to care for Sarah, maintaining her dignity and comfort until her death.

Sarah's situation, classified here as phase 3, also outlines a situation where further surgery and critical treatment were deemed to be futile (phase 2). In other words, surgery would not improve Sarah's condition; indeed, to undertake further surgery could be deemed unnecessary and irresponsible. The length of time a patient spends in each of the three phases will vary depending upon the individual patient and condition. For example, you could be working alongside your mentor, nursing a patient in phase 1 for several weeks before the patient recovers or deteriorates and moves into phase 2. Some patients, like Sarah, may move from phase 1 through to phase 3 very quickly, in a matter of hours (Coombs et al. 2012). The point to make is how quickly conditions can change and therefore decision making by intensive care staff needs to be equally prompt to reflect the changing dynamics.

Activity 7.4   *Critical thinking*

A seminal piece of research in 1979 by Molter identified that the three most important requirements of families whose relatives are in critical care are assurance, information and proximity. This identifies the family's need to feel cared for, informed and close to the patient.

As a nurse caring for Sarah and her family, how can you incorporate Molter's three requirements into your support for Sarah's family?

An outline answer is given at the end of this chapter.

In Activity 7.4 you might have identified areas like providing information to the family and allowing the family to visit at flexible times. These are all aspects of the care that is included once a patient is in phase 3 of the trajectory. The aim is to ensure comfort, peace and a dignified death. It is widely recognised that the majority of critically ill patients who are in phase 2 of the trajectory discussed above are unconscious (Curtis and Vincent 2010). However, the plan of care will be explained to patients, irrespective of their level of consciousness. It is known that hearing is the last sense to go when patients become unconscious, so it is important that health care professionals assume patients can still hear and communicate with them accordingly. This may involve both verbal and non-verbal communication – touch when talking to them and verbal communication to inform them what you are doing.

Nursing the dying patient in critical care

The design of a critical care unit cannot be underestimated in planning for space and private rooms for a grieving family. The design of critical care units varies across the UK. The number of beds, the layout, the number of single rooms and the number of beds in open spaces/bays will all differ. The physical limitations of critical care can prove challenging in maintaining dignity and support for the relatives when providing palliative and end of life care. A large open-area bay may be occupied by several critically ill patients, with each 'bed space' separated only by curtains for screening and privacy. If there is an available single room the patient may be moved from an open area to a single room to enable a greater level of privacy. However, this is not always possible as single rooms are frequently occupied by patients requiring isolation due to infection. Recognising the need for privacy at this time should be considered; curtains and screens can only provide so much privacy. Thompson et al. (2012) recommend that places off the critical care area should be made available so that a 'quiet space' is available for relatives. In most cases relatives can understand the physical limitations of the intensive care units, but staff need to reiterate this point to them as a way of acknowledging how difficult it might be for them not being close to the patient (loved one). This also enhances communication between staff and the relatives.

Removal of monitoring equipment

When active therapy is withdrawn the audible and visual alarm systems from the monitoring systems may be switched off. This might not always be the case; some critical care settings switch monitoring screens off and remove them from the bedside while others continue or reduce monitoring (McAree and Doherty 2010; Woodrow 2011). Removing equipment and machinery from the bedside seems to promote a peaceful and dignified setting for the patient and family. This action is congruent with Coombs et al.'s (2012) description of returning the person to the family, and it can present an almost tangible effect on the family becoming closer to the patient. In contrast to other health care settings, some patients may die within minutes or hours after active therapy is withdrawn. This can be influenced by factors such as the severity of organ failure and how dependent the patient was on supportive therapy. When the family are not at the bedside you may often see the nurse sitting with the patient and holding his or her hand (McCallum and McConigley 2013). This simple gesture, the use of therapeutic touch, supports the principle of ensuring a patient does not die alone.

Patients who are intubated and require ventilation continue to receive some respiratory support from a ventilator. However the percentage of oxygen being administered may be reduced. It is rare for a patient to be extubated (McAree and Doherty 2010); the overall aim of maintaining ventilator support is to avoid distressing the patient and to reduce dyspnoea.

Communication and palliative care in critical care

Case study

Steve's wife

I felt relief when the doctors and nurses talked to us about Steve. Going into the unit every day and seeing him there in the middle of all that technology trying to get him better . . . Time went by and all the treatment was tried but sometimes you have to just accept it . . . We talked through Steve's condition and the staff explained things. We felt the pressure was off us as the consultant described what was going to happen and also gave us some time to come to terms and make some plans. He had fought so hard but the sepsis was just too much . . .

Ensuring and maintaining excellent communication between staff and relatives is crucial when caring for the dying patient in critical care. The overwhelming nature of the setting and the situation can mean that conversations with relatives are forgotten or information is misunderstood. Some critical care units have customised 'communication sheets' in the patient notes covering meetings and updates for the family. In addition these will include information related to the withdrawal of active therapy in favour of palliation and end of life care (Intensive Care Society 2003). If you have experienced a practice placement in critical care you may have viewed notes either in an electronic or paper format. Documentation of meetings needs to be clear and consistent. Documentation should include the date and time of the meeting, names of staff and family present, the issues discussed and comments made by the family and staff. To improve communication between members of the health care team and with the relatives it is good practice for all meetings to include both a member of the nursing team and one of the doctors involved in the care of the patient. This ensures that members of the team are aware of what has been said to the family, can offer consistent support and can promote continuity of care between different shifts, including on-call staff.

Effective and supportive communication can support the family to ask questions and clarify any concerns they have. In addition the length of stay for the patient in critical care often influences the amount of information given and the development of rapport between staff and the patient's family and close friends. It is clearly acknowledged that you, as the nurse, are best placed to know the views of the relatives (Intensive Care Society 2003; Coombs and Long 2008; Coombs et al. 2012). The nurse caring for the dying patient will ascertain and document important information about the family and the patient to assist the plan of care. The information will include spiritual care and detail relating to family members wishing to be present at the bedside when death occurs.

Communication sheets (mentioned earlier) continue to be completed. Some critical care units have developed their own template related to withdrawal of active therapy in end of life care (Intensive Care Society 2003). Explicit sections of the notes provide an important log of events in relation to when meetings occur, what has been said by whom and what plans were proposed. A template or notes also promote continuity between the multidisciplinary team working shifts and on-call rotas. Although such practice happens in all nursing environments, in critical care it is important to keep these documents up to date as death can occur quite quickly.

Activity 7.5   *Evidence-based practice and research*

During your next practice placement take the time to visit the ITU or critical care unit in the hospital where you are working. Discuss with staff how palliative care is practised and what documentation is used to support palliative and end of life care in their setting.

As this activity is based on your own observations, there is no outline answer at the end of this chapter.

Whichever approach you find in Activity 7.5, the key aim must be for clear, precise communication with all involved and for all health care professionals to be familiar with the process. Currently there is variation in the documentation used and how the stages of end of life care are managed. Some critical care units have developed specific well-established NHS trust protocols or tools. Some follow broad principles of the national strategy (Department of Health 2008). Until 2013 one widely available framework was the Liverpool Care Pathway – intensive care unit process, known as LCP-ICU (MCPCIL 2011). The LCP-ICU was a useful tool, providing a clear structure that allowed care to be maintained and evaluated against measurable goals. However, at the time of writing a review of the LCP has recommended that it be phased out (see Chapter 6). As with any tool, it was as good or bad as the team using it, and whatever replaces the LCP should retain its positive aspects.

Involving the family in the care

Family members and friends whose relatives are receiving palliative and end of life care in a critical care setting often experience feelings of helplessness. They may want to be more actively involved in some of the practical aspects of the patient's care. The family may have already been involved in care during phase 1 (recovery) and phase 2 (transition) of active therapy. Family members can be involved in activities like assisting in administering mouth care, shaving and hair care. Support from you, by providing reassurance and expertise, will increase the relatives' confidence in carrying out these activities. As well as more practical activities, family members may like to play music or talk to the patient. If family members are unsure whether the dying person can hear them or not, always assume that the patient can hear. You will play an important role here in 'normalising' verbal communication with the patient, encouraging the family to talk naturally to the patient. Initially relatives may feel embarrassed and some members may be afraid to talk to the patient. By supporting relatives to talk to the patient you can assist the family to feel a 'connection' with him or her. Some family members may give simple updates of what is happening day to day in their community and others recognise it to be a time of saying goodbye and reminiscing about their time together. You should be sensitive to this need for privacy and take the time to physically 'stand back' from the bedside (Coombs et al. 2012).

Caring for yourself

The nurse-to-patient ratio of 1:1 or 1:2 in patient care in critical care reinforces the philosophy of holistic, patient-centred care. However, mortality rates are high, showing that palliative and end of life care can be a regular aspect of critical care nursing (Adam and Osborne 2005; Intensive Care National Audit and Research Centre 2010; Pattison et al. 2013).

Activity 7.6   *Reflection*

Reflect back on your answers to Activities 7.1 and 7.2 and answer the following questions:

- Did you consider that providing palliative and end of life care would feature regularly in a critical care setting? Why was that?
- Has your original view of critical care changed? If so, how?

As this activity is based on your own observations, there is no outline answer at the end of this chapter.

In your answer to Activity 7.6 you may have recognised the role that palliative and end of life care have in critical care and the impact of this on you. Doing this will encourage you to develop your knowledge and skills in this area. The other chapters in this book address many essential aspects of palliative and end of life care that you can use to support your care in a critical care setting. For example, Chapter 2 (Holistic patient care in palliative and end of life care) will support you to ensure that the essential care continues, e.g. ensuring comfort, pressure care, eye and mouth care and administration of medication for sedation and analgesia. Chapter 5 (Exploring the impact of culture issues in palliative and end of life care) will provide you with an understanding of how different people's beliefs influence their approach to death and dying. This can assist you to provide individual care where everyone is working in collaboration.

The most challenging phase for you, and other nurses, in critical care might be phase 2. When the decision to withdraw active treatment is made it is important that staff have confidence that everything was done for the patient and there is agreement in the decision making (McAree and Doherty 2010). You may not necessarily feel comfortable with the decision that has been made; however you need to have confidence that the decision was the right one and was in the best interest of the patient. This may result in some tension between members of the health care team. This is often the case if the nurse feels that the decision-making process was delayed and therapy prolonged (Walker and Read 2010; Coombs et al. 2012). It should be recognised that decisions cannot always be made quickly. Some patients may be cared for by several clinical speciality teams and a consensus needs to be reached by all these teams. The decision to withdraw active treatment is not an easy one to make; positive, open interdisciplinary team work can support staff to understand and accept the rationale for the decision. Due to the nurse's very visible role at the bedside, McCallum and McConigley (2013) describe the nurse as the protector of the patient, with the aim of promoting a peaceful, dignified death in what can be a noisy environment.

A key aspect in terms of your personal well-being and performance and in staff retention is to have a supportive positive team ethos. It is widely recognised that critical care nurses require ongoing education and clinical supervision to address end of life care (Adam and Osborne 2005; Stayt 2009; Walker and Read 2010; Shannon et al. 2011; Woodrow 2011). This can be done formally through ongoing staff development and clinical supervision. Additionally, having time to debrief, as a team, is important; this can be done informally or in a more structured manner. Having the time to reflect on the care provided, the decisions made and how palliative and end of life care was managed is crucial for the well-being of staff and the continuity of care for future patients. You and your colleagues will respond in different ways to the death of a patient. Scholes (2006) recalls a situation where a doctor sat distressed, head in hands, during the end of life care of a patient. The impact on the doctor was one of dismay and a feeling of failure in not facilitating recovery. Rather than reflect on 'watching them die' the nurses and the team can be 'with' the dying person, ensuring comfort and peace.

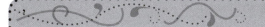

Chapter summary

This chapter has provided an overview of the role that palliative and end of life care has in a critical care setting. The three phases of care have been discussed and applied to case studies; the challenge presented by phase 2 has been recognised and explored in relation to providing palliative and end of life care. Strategies to support families have been outlined, including promoting communication and family involvement in the care of the patient. It is always important in any care you give to know yourself (self-awareness). Being aware of your feelings and values, and how you respond, will impact on the care that you provide for your patients. Some patients' values and beliefs may not reflect your own, but you may have to accept these as a professional caring for your patients. Finally, taking care of yourself, the role of peer support and clinical supervision have been identified as crucial and necessary to support you in providing palliative and end of life care for patients and their families.

Activities: brief outline answers

Activity 7.2: Reflection

Your search may have led you to specific NHS trust site units with an overview of information for patients and visitors. Hospitals may have a general intensive care unit where all seriously ill patients are admitted or they may have further specialities, e.g. neurosciences, trauma, liver and cardiothoracic. These critical care areas feature across the UK. Some units may differ depending on the type of patient admitted, e.g. a cardiothoracic unit has a higher incidence of elective patients specifically post heart and lung surgery and their stay in critical care is relatively short in comparison to a trauma or liver critical care unit where patients may have multiple medical complexities.

Activity 7.3: Critical thinking

You might have identified feelings of sadness, frustration and helplessness that there was no further treatment that could be provided for Tom. Recognising this and taking positive steps to address this is key to maintaining your well-being and promoting professional development. It may be helpful to express your feelings to your mentor or the qualified staff you are working alongside. Many nurses will automatically pick up your cues as to how you are feeling, and it can also help to talk to your peers about the challenges you face. Remember staff, just as much as families, need time to process their emotions.

It may be possible (although rare) that you feel that Tom would be at peace and not suffering anymore. You might have thought death was most appropriate given Tom's deteriorating condition. In that case you would still need to 'listen' to yourself and how you are feeling at the time. It is always important to care for yourself in both good and bad outcomes to care.

Activity 7.4: Critical thinking

Assurance – providing reassurance to Sarah's family, being realistic, not too pessimistic or unrealistically optimistic about the situation. Giving Sarah's family time to ask any questions, talk about their situation and ask them what concerns them.

Information – providing appropriate information to Sarah's family, how much information they want: some people might want to know everything, whereas others might only want to know a little at a time. Ensuring they understand the information that is being provided.

Proximity – explaining the equipment to Sarah's family, allowing them to sit by Sarah and to be physically close to her. Letting Sarah's family know that they can touch and talk to Sarah is also important in allowing Sarah's family to connect with her.

Further reading

Kongsuwan, W., Chaipetch, O. and Matchim Y. (2012) Thai Buddhist families' perspective of a peaceful death in ICUs. *Nursing in Critical Care*, 17 (3): 151–159.

This article outlines a qualitative study involving family members and their experience.

Ryder-Lewis, M. (2005) Going home from ICU to die: a celebration of life. *Nursing in Critical Care*, 10 (3): 116–121.

This article discusses the experience of one ICU department when supporting a dying patient to go home to die.

Stayt, L.C. (2009) Death, empathy and self-preservation: the emotional labour of caring for families of the critically ill in adult intensive care. *Journal of Clinical Nursing*, 18: 1267–1275.

A study of the impact on nurses supporting patients and their families in critical care and subsequent recommendations.

Useful websites

http://www.baccn.org.uk

The British Association of Critical Care Nurses promotes the art and science of critical care nursing. The Association works in collaboration in professional development and policy making.

http://www.gmc-uk.org/guidance/ethical_guidance/end_of_life_care.asp

This site provides information on *Treatment and care towards end of life: good practice in decision making* (2010) and includes information on withdrawing treatment.

http://www.ics.ac.uk/ics-homepage

This is the homepage for the Intensive Care Society. This body represents intensive care professionals and promotes the delivery of quality care for patients in critical care settings. Their guidelines and standards section has information on bereavement in critical care and other aspects of palliative and end of life care.

Chapter 8
Legal aspects of palliative and end of life care

Helen Taylor

NMC Standards for Pre-registration Nursing Education

This chapter will address the following competencies:

Domain 1: Professional values

1. All nurses must practice according to *The Code: Standards of Conduct, Performance and Ethics for Nurses and Midwives* (NMC 2008), and within other recognised ethical and legal frameworks. They must be able to recognise and address ethical challenges relating to people's choices and decision making about their care, and act within the law to help them and their families and carers find acceptable solutions.
2. All nurses must practise in a holistic, non-judgemental, caring and sensitive manner that avoids assumptions; supports social inclusion; recognises and respects individual choice; and acknowledges diversity. Where necessary, they must challenge inequality, discrimination and exclusion from care.

NMC Essential Skills Clusters

This chapter will address the following:

Cluster: Organisational aspects of care

11. People can trust the newly registered graduate nurse to safeguard children and adults from vulnerable situations and support and protect them from harm.

First progression point

1. Acts within legal frameworks and local policies in relation to safeguarding adults and children who are in vulnerable situations.

By the second progression point

4. Documents concerns and information about people who are in vulnerable situations.

Entry to the register

9. Supports people in asserting their human rights.
10. Challenges practices which do not safeguard those in need of support and protection.

Chapter aims

After reading this chapter you will be able to:

- explore the legal basis of a nurse's obligation to provide patient care;
- appreciate the importance of patient autonomy;
- explain the law in relation to consent and refusal to consent;
- reflect on legal issues relating to the sanctity of life;
- evaluate and define circumstances where treatment may lawfully be withdrawn or withheld.

Introduction

Scenarios

Imagine that you find yourself in one of these two situations.

Matthew has been admitted to your ward with a chest infection; it is his third admission in less than two months. He is 13 years old and has cystic fibrosis, and is awaiting a lung transplant. You go to see him shortly before his infusion of intravenous antibiotics is due to commence. As you approach the bed you notice that Matthew is crying. You sit down and ask him what is wrong. He replies that 'everything is wrong' and that he has 'had enough'. You hold his hand in a supportive way until he stops crying. At that point he tells you that, although his parents are desperate for him to receive new lungs, he has decided that he does not want to go through with it, nor does he want to continue with treatment for his current infection.

Claire is 54 years old and has early-onset Alzheimer's disease. She is admitted to your unit with a severe chest infection, and currently appears confused and disorientated. She is accompanied by her partner, Anna, who tells you that Claire 'hates how she is'. Anna tells you that, before Claire's condition deteriorated, they often discussed the future and how Claire would prefer to manage her condition. Anna tells you that Claire was aware that in time she would lose the ability to care for herself and make her own decisions. Anna tells you that Claire would want you to 'just let her go' and not treat the infection.

Activity 8.1   *Reflection*

Now, think about how you might respond to Matthew, Claire and Anna.

- How confident would you feel in these circumstances?
- Why?
- What are your learning needs?

> *Brief answers to all activities are given at the end of the chapter, unless otherwise indicated. This activity is based on your own observations, so there is no outline answer given.*

Undertaking the reflection in Activity 8.1 will provide you with a baseline in relation to your knowledge and confidence regarding legal aspects of palliative care. This chapter will support you to develop your knowledge and confidence relating to legal issues in palliative and end of life care. No consideration of end of life care would be complete without exploring the impact of law on the delivery of care, for example, issues relating to consent to treatment and an individual's capacity to consent. However, whilst consent is a matter to be considered for all patients, regardless of their health status and general condition, there are some legal issues that relate only to those approaching the end of their lives, for example, the withholding of life-sustaining treatment.

You will be aware of the professional, public and media focus during 2013 on the Liverpool Care Pathway. This has highlighted a deep sense of unease at what, in some cases, has appeared to be arbitrary withdrawal of even the most basic of human needs such as nutrition and hydration. This increased attention to often very difficult decisions associated with end of life care has culminated in an independent review of the Liverpool Care Pathway. This review recommended that this generic protocol for the care of the dying be replaced with individualised plans of care, supported by practice guidelines (Independent Review of the Liverpool Care Pathway 2013).

However, the fact remains that, when a dying person is no longer able to tolerate oral fluids, there is no requirement in law to administer even subcutaneous fluids if this is not in the patient's best interests (Independent Review of the Liverpool Care Pathway 2013). Many people find this difficult to accept or understand. Even in situations where the Liverpool Care Pathway has been carefully and appropriately implemented, there is no doubt that some health care professionals experience a sense of discomfort when attempts at curative treatments and even basic life support end. It is counterintuitive: from the moment you embarked on your career, the instinct is to act to preserve life. How can it be that on the one hand it may be permissible, and entirely appropriate, to discontinue intravenous infusion of fluids, whilst on the other it would be unlawful to administer an intramuscular injection of diamorphine with the intention of terminating someone's life, regardless of how much pain that person is suffering?

This chapter will give you the opportunity to understand how the law applies in a variety of end of life care scenarios.

Obligation to treat

Before going on to consider the law as it relates specifically to end of life care, it is very important that you understand some fundamental legal issues. For example, there are a number of categories of law, but the two that this chapter will focus on are criminal and civil law. These two areas of law have some significant differences. For example, the aim of criminal law is to impose state requirements for the conduct of its citizens in order to maintain order and enable public protection, whilst the aim of civil law is to enforce obligations (e.g. contract, trespass and negligence) between individuals and/or organisations. A breach of the criminal law may result in an action being brought by the state, and if a prosecution is successful, punishments such as imprisonment, fines, community orders, rehabilitation orders, and many more, may be imposed. Conversely, an action for breach of civil law can be brought by any individual or organisation affected by the breach, and if successful may result in compensation being awarded for any loss resulting from this breach (Slapper and Kelly 2013).

Negligence (civil law – negligence)

The primary focus of this chapter will be on civil law – the obligations that exist between an individual (or organisation) and other individuals (or organisations). These legal responsibilities may arise in a number of ways. For example, if you enter into a contract with a builder for him to build you a new extension for £20,000, you will have a legal obligation to pay him £20,000 when he builds it. In turn, the builder will be required to build your extension as specified in the contract. Similarly, if you buy a holiday from a travel company, they must ensure that the holiday provided is as described. In these two examples the obligations arise from a clearly recognisable and formal contract, with much of the detail of each party's obligations specified either verbally or in writing. Sometimes, however, civil law obligations do not come from any form of written or verbal contract, but arise from a particular situation rather than any formally recognised relationship (Halsbury's Laws of England 2010a). This area of civil law is known as *tort*, and one example is negligence, as explained by Lord Aitkin in *Donoghue* v *Stevenson* ([1932] p580):

> *You must take reasonable care to avoid acts or omissions which you can reasonably foresee would be likely to injure your neighbour. Who then, in law is my neighbour? The answer seems to be – persons who are so closely and directly affected by my act that I ought reasonably to have them in contemplation as being so affected when I am directing my mind to the acts or omissions which are called into question.*

By recognising the possibility that an individual (you do not even need to know who the person is) or a general group of people could be affected by your actions or failure to act, you have established a duty of care to these people – your 'neighbours' in law. Your response will be judged against the standard of the 'reasonable person' – a legal test which considers 'is this what a reasonable person either would or would not have done?' (*Blyth* v *Birmingham Waterworks* [1856]). This means that you have a legal responsibility to ensure that your acts, or omissions, do not cause harm to anyone who you could reasonably anticipate being affected by your actions, or failure to act, in a particular situation.

A useful way of summarising the application of the general law of negligence is to ask yourself:

1. Does a duty of care exist?
2. Has it been breached (either by doing something or failing to do something that a reasonable person would either have done or not done)?
3. Has harm been suffered?
4. Is this harm of a type that is reasonably foreseeable?

If you answer yes to each of these questions, you may be liable in negligence.

> **Scenario**
>
> *You are coming towards the end of a busy day in practice, and still have a long list of things that you would like to complete before you go home. As you rush away from the nurses' station you knock over a mug of coffee that someone had left. The mug does not break, but some coffee spills on to the corridor. You deliberate for a moment but decide that you will come back later to mop up the spillage.*

Although you intend to return and clean up the coffee later, by leaving it, there is a risk that colleagues, patients or visitors to the ward might slip on the spillage and injure themselves. By creating a potentially dangerous situation (spilling the drink) you have established a duty of care to people likely to be affected by this – other individuals using the corridor. Most reasonable people would ensure that the drink was mopped up in order to remove the hazard. If you did not do that, you breached your duty of care to other people passing along the corridor. If someone were to slip and sustain an injury (which could reasonably be foreseen as the result of slipping on a hard floor), then you might be liable in negligence.

Activity 8.2   *Decision making*

Apply the test of negligence in these situations. On the evidence provided, do you think there may be liability in negligence?

1. Martin is sitting in the busy reception area of the university. He is eating a banana whilst reading this book. He is so eager to finish reading this chapter that, rather than putting the banana skin in the nearby waste bin, he throws it on to the floor behind him and hopes that no one notices. Simon is on his way to a lecture and does not see the banana skin and slips on it. Unfortunately he suffers a fractured wrist as a result. He loses his part-time job as a waiter, and is not able to play rugby for the rest of the season.
2. You decide to take a break from your studies by going for a relaxing walk in the countryside. You cross a field full of cows, and walk through a gateway on to a winding lane. You do not close the gate behind you, and the cows escape into the lane. Emma is also taking a break from work, but has decided to go on a cycle ride. She rounds a bend and is met by the herd of cattle that have escaped from the field that you failed to secure by closing the gate. Emma is unable to stop her bike safely and falls, fracturing her collar bone and damaging her bike. The cows stampede and a number suffer injuries. The farmer's fence is also damaged.

An outline answer is given at the end of this chapter.

Clinical negligence

The previous examples of negligence come from daily life, but for you, as a health care professional, special rules apply. It is usually quite a straightforward task to establish that nurses and other health care professionals not only have a civil law duty of care for their patients, but must also exercise reasonable skill in providing this care (Halsbury's Laws of England 2011a).

There is a wide body of case law which explores and defines this. For example, the case of *Cassidy* v *Ministry of Health* ([1951] p360), where Lord Denning made clear his opinion on the responsibilities of health care providers:

> [A]uthorities who run a hospital, be they local authorities, government boards, or any other corporation, are in law under the self-same duty as the humblest doctor; whenever they accept a patient for treatment, they must use reasonable care and skill to cure him of his ailment. The hospital authorities cannot, of course, do it by themselves: they have no ears to listen through the stethoscope, and no hands to hold the surgeon's knife. They must do it by the staff which they employ; and if their staff are negligent in giving the treatment, they are just as liable for that negligence as is anyone else who employs others to do his duties for him. What possible difference in law, I ask, can there be between hospital authorities who accept a patient for treatment, and railway or shipping authorities who accept a passenger for carriage? None whatever. Once they undertake the task, they come under a duty to use care in the doing of it, and that is so whether they do it for reward or not.

So, unlike general negligence, the boundaries (parameters) of clinical negligence are more clearly defined. For example, in a therapeutic relationship (unlike in general negligence) there is unlikely to be much debate about the existence of a duty of care between you and your patient. Also, the standard of care will likely be higher. The test will not be the standard exercised by the 'reasonable person', but instead you will be judged against other nurses with the same education, training and skills.

Quite how this might be determined is a question that has been explored and debated at great length. However, the general position in law is still provided by a case that was decided more than 50 years ago in *Bolam* v *Friern Management Committee* ([1957] p122), where McNair, J., stated that *a doctor is not guilty of negligence if he has acted in accordance with a practice accepted as proper by a responsible body of medical men skilled in that particular art.*

Over the intervening years this test, now widely known as the 'Bolam test', has been subject to further refinement and clarification. In essence this means that the standard of care can now be more generally applied to all health care professionals, including nurses, and will be measured against what is regarded as reasonable and logical (*Bolitho* v *City and Hackney H.A.* [1997]) at the time the act or omission in question took place.

At this point it is worth mentioning that those working for organisations which sit outside the National Health Service – for example, private hospitals and care agencies – may also be subject to legislation which regulates the provision of purchased services, such as the Supply of Goods and Services Act 1982. However, regardless of the source of the law, there is an expectation that nurses will provide care of a reasonable standard. This is in addition to the ethical and professional imperatives considered in Chapter 6 that will ensure that patients receive end of life care that is not only evidence-based, person-centred and of good quality. Activity 8.3 will prompt you to apply your critical thinking and problem-solving skills to your knowledge of legal issues.

Read again the preceding paragraphs and think carefully about patients reaching the end of their life. Consider the words of Lord Denning, and make a note of any questions that come to your mind in response to his statement.

At the end of the chapter you should return to your list of questions and see how many remain unanswered. Now, as a critical health care professional, your next task is to undertake further reading and investigation to answer those outstanding questions. The further reading at the end of the chapter is a good starting point.

As this activity is based on your own observations, there is no outline answer at the end of this chapter.

Consent in palliative and end of life care

Having read the previous section you will have noticed that the emphasis is very much on the role and responsibilities of both the health care provider (such as the hospital or hospice) and individual nurses and other health care professionals. One very important member of the care relationship has yet to be considered, and that of course is the patient. It is all very well to talk about the imperative to deliver good-quality care, but that completely disregards any recognition of patients' rights to involvement in decisions about their care. Although health care providers and professionals have a civil law obligation to make an offer of care, patients are generally under no legal obligation to accept that offer.

'Consent' is a word used widely in health care; voluntary provision of valid and informed consent is generally recognised as a necessary part of treatment. But why is consent so important?

Think about some of the situations where you have witnessed a patient giving consent and reflect on the following:

- What was the patient consenting to? Did the patient know? Can you be sure of that? How?
- Did you know what the patient was consenting to? Did you need to know?
- How did the patient communicate consent? Was it always in the same way?
- Is it important that consent is given in the same way? Why?
- Were there any situations where treatment was given without the patient being asked for consent? Why? What did you think about that? Why?

As this activity is based on your own observations, there is no outline answer at the end of this chapter.

Activity 8.4 allowed you to reflect on the importance of consent and what it means to the therapeutic relationship between you and your patients. The importance of a patient giving voluntary, informed consent before receiving any form of treatment or therapeutic intervention is underpinned by the ethical and legal principle of self-determination (see Chapter 6 for a discussion of the ethics). Lord Goff stated: *The fundamental principle, plain and incontestable, is that every person's body is inviolate* (*Collins* v *Wilcock* [1984] p378). This means that we all have the right to decide who touches our body, and that any touching without our consent is generally unlawful. This principle is so important that unusually, touching without consent (referred to in law as 'battery') will constitute a breach of both criminal and civil law. Even putting someone in fear of non-consensual touching is unlawful, and is known as an 'assault' (Halsbury's Laws of England 2010b).

This terminology can be confusing, but because 'assault' is usually synonymous with 'battery', the general tendency is to adopt the term 'assault' for both offences (*Fagan* v *Metropolitan Police Commissioner* [1968]), and you will often hear the offence referred to as 'common assault'. Although both crimes originated from the common law, they are now enshrined in s39 of the Criminal Justice Act 1988 and constitute summary offences punishable by a level 5 fine of up to £5,000 (the maximum level on the standard scale prescribed by Criminal Justice Act 1982 (as amended) s37) and/or a prison sentence of up to six months.

Consent therefore serves as a legal defence – a legal 'safety blanket' that makes lawful what would otherwise be unlawful. There are some other defences to assault and battery, such as self-defence; prevention of crime; protection of property and the lawful chastisement of a child, but further consideration of these is not necessary for the purpose of this chapter. Without valid consent, any touching of a patient's body will therefore be unlawful. Other than in some exceptional circumstances (which will be detailed below) consent is required before any treatment or therapeutic intervention can lawfully take place.

What is valid consent?

As identified in your reflection in Activity 8.4, consent will only be valid if it has been freely given by a fully informed person who has the capacity to make that decision. Patients must be told both the risks and the benefits associated with the proposed treatment or intervention (*Chester* v *Afshar* [2004]), be able to evaluate that information and then communicate their decision.

The rules regarding decision-making capacity differ for children, young adults and adults. The Mental Capacity Act 2005 has enshrined in statute the presumption that adults and young people aged 16 years and older (further to s8 Family Law Reform Act 1969) will have decision-making capacity unless they have some permanent or temporary *impairment of, or a disturbance in the functioning of, the mind or brain* (Mental Capacity Act 2005, s2 (1)) which renders them unable to make a decision about a particular issue. The position for children aged under 16 is different. The case of *Gillick* v *West Norfolk and Wisbech AHA* [1986] established that children *may* have capacity to consent to treatment, providing that they fully understand the implications both of having and not having the treatment, and are able to demonstrate that they can both recall this information and make their decision known (General Medical Council 2007).

If the patient lacks decision-making capacity (according to the provisions of the Mental Capacity Act 2005), treatment may still be given providing:

- it is in the patient's best interests (Mental Capacity Act 2005, s (5)), and
- the patient has not made a valid advance decision refusing that treatment (Mental Capacity Act 2005, s (24)).

It may sometimes be necessary for the court to make an order that treatment would be in the patient's interests and may therefore go ahead lawfully:

> *The substantive law is that a proposed operation is lawful if it is in the best interests of the patient, and unlawful if it is not. What is required from the court, therefore, is not an order giving approval to the operation, so as to make lawful that which would otherwise be unlawful. What is required from the court is rather an order which establishes by judicial process . . . whether the proposed operation is in the best interests of the patient and therefore lawful, or not in the patient's best interests and therefore unlawful.*
>
> (Lord Oakbrook in *F v West Berkshire Health Authority (Mental Health Act Commission intervening)* [1989] p557)

The test of best interests will be the *Bolam test,* as considered previously in the section on clinical negligence, above.

Refusal of consent

If an adult (over 18 years in the UK) with decision-making capacity refuses consent, then treatment may not go ahead, even if those caring for that patient consider the patient's decision to be foolish or irrational or the refusal results in the patient's death (for example, *Re T (An Adult: Refusal of Medical Treatment)* [1992]). This may be very difficult for health care professionals to accept, but it is so important to acknowledge the right to self-determination that sometimes this must even supersede *the principle of sanctity of human life* (Lord Goff in *Airedale NHS Trust v Bland* [1993] p866).

For children and young adults (those aged between 16 and 18 years) the position is different. Providing they have decision-making capacity they may consent to treatment, even if their parents (or those with parental responsibility for them) do not consent to the treatment. However, if the child or young person refuses to consent, then the treatment may lawfully go ahead providing their parents, those with parental responsibility or the Court do consent (*Re W (A Minor) (Medical Treatment: Court's Jurisdiction)* [1992]).

Activity 8.5	*Reflection*

Think about the previous paragraphs relating to refusal of consent. Have you ever been in a situation where a patient has refused to consent to treatment?

- How did this make you feel at the time? Were you tempted/did you attempt to make the patient change his or her mind?
- How do you think the patient felt about his or her decision?
- What makes you think that? Why do you think the patient made that decision?

continued ... •

- How did the patient's family and friends respond?
- What impact did this refusal have on your care of the patient?
- How did the matter conclude?
- How would you manage a situation like this in the future?

As this activity is based on your own observations, there is no outline answer at the end of this chapter.

In reflecting on Activity 8.5, you may have considered how difficult it is for health care professionals to accept a patient's decision to refuse treatment, e.g. when they know that treatment will relieve a patient's pain. Therefore, it is possible that professionals may try to influence the patient to change his or her decision. Some family members may want treatment regardless, as they truly believe it will save the patient's life. There are many other ways of analysing this, but what is important in all this is to do what is best for the patient – to act in the best interest of the patient.

Legal consideration of the sanctity of life

When individuals approach the end of their life, they may not be able to fulfil their holistic care needs. Their illness may bring with it severe pain, cognitive decline or other symptoms that make it difficult for them either to engage with or enjoy their usual daily activities. Their family and friends may find it increasingly difficult to watch the person they love deteriorate and possibly suffer.

For some patients you may find that symptom management is difficult, and patients find their condition intolerable. In situations such as this, some people may ask: 'Is a life like this worth living?' This is a difficult question and confronts one of the fundamental principles of our society – that human life is sacred, and should be protected at all costs.

Activity 8.6	*Critical thinking*

Peter is 49 years old, and is married with two teenaged children. Despite never having smoked, Peter was diagnosed with lung cancer early last year. Before becoming unwell, Peter had been fit and well, combining his love of marathon running with his job as an engineer, and being – as described by his wife – 'the best dad and husband anyone could hope for'. Since his diagnosis, Peter has received a range of treatments, including chemotherapy, and he was distressed by how ill this made him. For a time he appeared to improve, but recently his condition has deteriorated. Sadly, he has been advised that his condition is now terminal, and that there is no prospect of a cure. He has been offered further chemotherapy in an attempt to prolong his life, and has been advised that, without it, his life expectancy is likely to be less than two months. Peter was very distressed by this news, but has decided that he would rather make the most of his final weeks away from the hospital and with his loved ones.

Now, imagine that Peter is one of your patients and consider the following questions:

- How do you feel about this decision? How easy is it to accept Peter's decision?
- What might be the impact on Peter's family?
- How might it affect Peter's relationship with his family?
- What is the potential effect on Peter's relationship with members of care staff?
- What is your role in supporting Peter and his family?

As this activity is based on your own observations, there is no outline answer at the end of this chapter.

The taking, or otherwise prematurely bringing to the end, of a life is taboo and considered so abhorrent that our society reserves its most severe sanctions for those who breach it. A conviction for murder, for example – where the accused intended to kill or very seriously injure – brings with it a mandatory sentence of life imprisonment. Even where someone caused death without intending to do so and is found guilty of manslaughter, the court may still impose a sentence of life imprisonment.

In your reflection in Activity 8.6 your patient was able to make an informed decision regarding refusing ongoing medical treatment. The case of *Airedale NHS Trust* v *Bland* [1993] required the House of Lords (at that time the highest Court of Appeal, a role subsequently assumed by the Supreme Court in 2009: Slapper and Kelly 2013) to consider some challenging questions relating to withdrawing treatment, the sanctity of life and the lawfulness of acting in any way other than to preserve life for a person who was not able to make an informed decision about ongoing medical treatment.

Case study

Anthony Bland was 17 years old when he was involved in what has come to be known as the 'Hillsborough disaster'. He was a Liverpool FC supporter and, on 15 April 1989, had travelled to the Hillsborough football ground for a semifinal of the FA Cup between Liverpool FC and Nottingham Forest FC. More than 90 supporters of both teams died after a catastrophic crush developed. Anthony received serious injuries to his chest, and as a result his brain was deprived of oxygen, resulting in severe injury.

By the autumn of 1992 Anthony had been in what was then known as a 'persistent vegetative state' (PVS) for more than three years, with no prospect of recovery (this is now more generally referred to as a vegetative state (VS): Airedale NHS Trust v Bland [1993]; W (by her litigation friend B) v M (by her litigation friend the Official Solicitor) and others [2011]). His condition meant that, although he could breathe without assistance, all higher-level brain functions had been permanently destroyed. Anthony had no sensory or cognitive awareness, and other than breathing, he required assistance with every bodily function. He was fed via a nasogastric tube.

Both the doctors treating Anthony and his family were of the opinion that it was inappropriate for his treatment to continue. The health authority made an application to the court for a declaration that

continued ...

> *withdrawal of all life-sustaining support (including artificial ventilation, hydration and nutrition)*
> *could be done lawfully so that Mr Bland could die as peacefully and with as much dignity as possible.*
> *At first instance the judge granted the declarations, but the Official Solicitor appealed, arguing that*
> *a withdrawal of treatment breached the doctors' duty of care to Mr Bland and would also incur*
> *criminal liability.*

The final appeal by Airedale NHS Trust was heard at the House of Lords in December 1992, and
a number of fundamental issues were considered, including:

- Must a patient's life be preserved by all medical means, regardless of the circumstances?
- What is the difference between an act that will hasten death and withdrawal of life-sustaining
  treatment?

This case is certainly tragic, and the report is deeply moving, but provides very useful clarification
in a number of key areas.

Activity 8.7 *Critical thinking*

Read this section of Lord Goff's judgement (*Airedale NHS Trust* v *Bland* [1993] pp873–874)
and, before reading the next section of this chapter, summarise the points raised:

> *[A]rtificial feeding is, in a case such as the present, no different from life support by a ven-*
> *tilator, and as such can lawfully be discontinued when it no longer fulfils any therapeutic*
> *purpose. To me, the crucial point in which I found myself differing from Mr Munby* [bar-
> rister acting for the Official Solicitor, and opposing the withdrawal of treatment] *was that I was unable to accept his treating the discontinuance of artificial feeding in the*
> *present case as equivalent to cutting a mountaineer's rope, or severing the air pipe of a deep*
> *sea diver. Once it is recognised, as I believe it must be, that the true question is not whether*
> *the doctor should take a course in which he will actively kill his patient, but rather whether*
> *he should continue to provide his patient with medical treatment or care which, if continued,*
> *will prolong his life, then, as I see it, the essential basis of Mr Munby's submissions disappears.*

Now read this earlier section (*Airedale NHS Trust* v *Bland* [1993] p868) and, before reading
the next section of this chapter, summarise the points raised here:

> *The doctor who is caring for such a patient cannot, in my opinion, be under an absolute*
> *obligation to prolong his life by any means available to him, regardless of the quality of*
> *the patient's life. Common humanity requires otherwise, as do medical ethics and good*
> *medical practice accepted in this country and overseas. As I see it, the doctor's decision*
> *whether or not to take any such step must (subject to his patient's ability to give or with-*
> *hold his consent) be made in the best interests of the patient. It is this principle too which,*
> *in my opinion, underlies the established rule that a doctor may, when caring for a patient*
> *who is, for example, dying of cancer, lawfully administer painkilling drugs despite the*
> *fact that he knows that an incidental effect of that application will be to abbreviate the*

> *patient's life. Such a decision may properly be made as part of the care of the living patient, in his best interests; and, on this basis, the treatment will be lawful. Moreover, where the doctor's treatment of his patient is lawful, the patient's death will be regarded in law as exclusively caused by the injury or disease to which his condition is attributable.*
> (*Airedale NHS Trust* v *Bland* [1993] p868)
>
> *A summary of the points will be given in the next section of this chapter.*

In relation to the judgement in Activity 8.7, the House of Lords provided some important clarification. You may have identified some of these when completing the activity:

1. Artificially administered hydration and nutrition are treatments and may lawfully be withdrawn or withheld if:

   a. they are no longer serving a therapeutic purpose or
   b. would no longer serve a therapeutic purpose and
   c. this would be in the patient's best interests.

2. If withdrawing or withholding artificial hydration and nutrition results in the shortening of a patient's life, then it is not the withdrawal of treatment that will have caused the death, but the underlying condition – for example, cancer or severe brain injury.

3. Such a withdrawal of treatment is regarded very differently in law to any act such as an overdose of analgesia that is deliberately intended either to end life or hasten death. This would be an unlawful killing.

4. However, it may be lawful to administer analgesia that is intended to act as palliative symptom control, even if an associated effect of this is to shorten the patient's life.

5. There is no legal obligation to continue treatment where the quality of a patient's life is poor and there is no prospect of recovery.

Careful reading of these points should help you to understand the legal principles underpinning guidelines for end of life care. The law does not provide for indiscriminate withdrawal, but instead makes very clear that feeding or hydration by artificial means should end only when they are providing no therapeutic purpose and to do so would be in the patient's best interests.

Each case should be considered on an individual basis, and the House of Lords ruled that consideration of best interests will usually require that treatment is given. However, respect must be given to the principle of self-determination. Where a patient has decision-making capacity the patient may refuse to consent to any treatment:

> *for any reason, rational or irrational, or for no reason at all, even where that decision may lead to his or her own death.*
> (*Re MB (Medical Treatment)* [1997] p432)

This means that, even where health care professionals consider a potentially life-saving treatment to be in a patient's best interests, providing the patient has capacity, the patient is under no obligation to accept that treatment.

Airedale NHS Trust v *Bland* [1993] predated the Mental Capacity Act 2005, and the provisions of this Act now shape the decision-making process for patients who no longer have decision-making capacity. You will recall the test for determining decision-making capacity from earlier in this chapter, and that there will be a presumption of decision-making capacity unless there is proof to the contrary (Mental Capacity Act 2005). So, assuming that the necessary assessment of capacity has been performed, and it has been concluded that your patient does not have capacity, how are treatment decisions at the end of life made?

Decision making in end of life care where patients lack capacity

Where the patient lacks decision-making capacity, there are a number of alternative ways in which decisions can be made on the patient's behalf. The patient may have made a valid advance decision to refuse a specified treatment should the need for it arise when the patient no longer has capacity to make decisions (Mental Capacity Act 2005, s24). If health care professionals reasonably believe that an applicable and valid advance decision to refuse treatment exists, they will be protected from legal liability for withdrawing or withholding treatment (for example, breach of duty in negligence). However, a number of conditions must be satisfied for a valid advance decision to refuse treatment (Department for Constitutional Affairs 2007):

1. The person making the advance decision (you may also see this referred to as an 'advance directive') must have mental capacity and be aged 18 or over at the time the decision was made.
2. The decision must specify treatment that the individual would like to refuse at a point when he or she no longer has decision-making capacity.
3. The decision must specify details of the treatment and the circumstances in which the patient would like to refuse it.
4. Any decision to refuse life-sustaining treatment must be in writing (make clear that the decision must still stand even if that individual's life is at risk), be signed and witnessed.

It is important to note that, whilst there is legal provision for patients to refuse treatment in advance, other than an obligation for professionals to respect (where possible) the patient's previously stated preferences (*Aintree University Hospitals NHS Foundation Trust* v *James* [2013]), there is generally no allied right to demand treatment in advance (*R (on the application of Burke)* v *General Medical Council* [2005]).

In addition to, or instead of, an advance directive, patients may have created a lasting power of attorney (LPA) (Mental Capacity Act 2005, s10) giving another person authority to make decisions on their behalf once they have lost the capacity to make decisions. Although there is no facility for patients to specify what treatment they would choose should they lose capacity, this is something that they would have discussed with their LPA(s). The LPA(s) should use that information to guide decision making on behalf of the patient who no longer has capacity. The Court of Protection also has authority under the Mental Capacity Act (2005, s16) to appoint a deputy to make decisions for a patient who does not have capacity.

In the absence of all of these, doctors may provide any treatment they consider to be in the patient's best interests (Mental Capacity Act 2005, s5). If there is any disagreement between medical opinion and the views of the patient's family and friends, the usual course of action is for the hospital to apply to the Court of Protection for a declaration that the proposed treatment can go ahead (Mental Capacity Act 2005, s15). Any decision will be made in the patient's interests, and should as far as possible take into account what is known of the patient's wishes whilst he or she had capacity.

Other issues deliberated by the House of Lords in the case of *Airedale NHS Trust* v *Bland* [1993] included the principle of the sanctity of human life. It was held that there is no obligation to preserve a patient's life by medical means, regardless of the individual circumstances. Indeed, in Lord Goff's opinion, the withdrawal of medical support, such as artificial nutrition, hydration and ventilation, should be considered in the same way as any other medical treatment. If continuing with the treatment is no longer in the patient's best interests (see the section below to learn more about determining a patient's best interests), then it will not be a breach of duty to discontinue treatment (this summary refers to lines 1–4 of Lord Goff's judgement, as referred to in Activity 8.7 on page 148).

Lord Goff went on to clarify the law in relation to discontinuing medical treatment that is no longer in the patient's best interests. He asserted that this is fundamentally different to committing an act with the intention of shortening a patient's life (this summary refers to lines 5–12 of Lord Goff's judgement, as referred to in Activity 8.7 on page 148), which would be unlawful. Therefore administration of medication with the intention of relieving pain would be lawful, even if it does have the secondary effect of shortening the patient's life. However, administration of analgesia with the intention of hastening death would be unlawful. The key difference is the intention behind the act.

The House of Lords made it clear that a decision to discontinue treatment could only be made after very careful consideration, and that a declaration from the Court of Protection would be necessary before artificial hydration or nutrition could lawfully be withheld or withdrawn from a patient in a VS. Since then, more recent guidance on applications for discontinuing treatment were issued by the Court of Protection in the case of *W (by her litigation friend B)* v *M (by her litigation friend the Official Solicitor) and others* [2011], to be referred to as: *W* v *M* 2011.

Case study

W v *M* [2011]

In February 2003 Mary was aged 43 and she became unwell at home the night before she was due to go on a skiing trip with her partner, Simon. She complained of a headache and went to bed early. Simon discovered her in a drowsy and confused state. Mary quickly deteriorated and was taken to hospital, where she was found to be suffering from viral encephalitis. She went into a coma, and when she eventually emerged, was diagnosed as being in a VS as the result of extensive and permanent brain damage continued ...

caused by the virus. From that point she required 24-hour assistance with all her needs, was doubly incontinent, and since April 2003 had been fed via a gastrostomy tube. Mary was also immobile. By the end of 2006, clinicians treating her at a specialist rehabilitation unit were of the view that there was unlikely to be any further improvement in her condition. By the time the case was heard in 2011, Mary had flexion contractures in the ankles, knees, hips and elbows.

On 16 January 2007, Mary's family and Simon made an application to the High Court Family Division for a ruling that Mary lacked capacity to make decisions about her medical care, and that it would be lawful to withhold and discontinue all life-sustaining treatment, including artificial hydration and nutrition. Although Simon reported that Mary had discussed with him the issue of ongoing treatment in such a situation, she had not written an advance directive, and there was no other evidence to support this.

Over the next two or three years there were a number of assessments of Mary's level of consciousness. Although she was initially thought to be in a VS, subsequent review by another expert suggested that her level of consciousness was higher than originally thought. In fact, her condition better fitted the criteria for someone in a minimally conscious state (MCS) rather than VS, and with intensive rehabilitation it was thought that Mary might recover further. However, despite five months of intensive rehabilitation, she failed to make any further improvement and did not demonstrate any high-level functional responses to her environment.

She was admitted to a nursing home in February 2008. At this point, and as part of the ongoing legal process, Mary was assessed again by a different expert. This assessment found that, although her condition was variable, there was no evidence that any aspect of Mary's life gave her satisfaction, pleasure, discomfort or pain. This new assessment placed Mary at the lowest end of MCS. It was the expert's opinion that it would be appropriate to withdraw life-sustaining treatment in order that Mary might die with dignity. Mary's family therefore decided to continue with the application, which was transferred to the new Court of Protection in February 2010. The two experts assessing Mary agreed that she remained in an MCS, with her responses less consistent than they had been previously. However, they disagreed over the question of withdrawing artificial hydration and nutrition.

In order to protect confidentiality, only initials are given in the case report. 'Mary' and 'Simon' are pseudonyms.

It is clear from the case report that over the years Mary and Simon had shared conversations about their wishes should they find themselves in such a tragic situation. Unfortunately the couple never formalised their conversations by making a valid, written advance decision. So, although Simon could use these discussions to help guide Mary's day-to-day care, it was not sufficient to allow a withdrawal of artificial hydration and nutrition. Therefore, given Mary's lack of capacity, and the absence of a valid advance decision, the Court was required to determine whether it was in Mary's best interests (as per s4 Mental Capacity Act 2005) to withdraw and withhold all life-sustaining treatment, including artificial nutrition and hydration (*W* v *M* [2011]).

In order to establish what was in Mary's best interests, the court adopted a balance sheet approach that had been advocated in an earlier case (*Re A (Medical Treatment: Male Sterilisation)* [2000]). This approach evaluated the advantages of withdrawing treatment as opposed to continuing with it, taking into consideration factors other than those that are purely medical, including *emotional and other welfare issues* (*Re A* [2000] p2000). The court also addressed a historic debate about the issue of 'intolerability', and whether that benchmark must be met before considering withdrawal of artificial hydration and nutrition to be in the patient's best interests. However, the view was that, rather than being a prerequisite for withdrawal of artificial hydration and nutrition, this should instead be considered as part of the balance sheet approach (*W v M* [2011]). The court also took into account how Mary's experience of life would be affected by necessary treatment (*NHS Trust v S* [2003] p47) and other requirements, as per s4 Mental Capacity Act 2005, and the Mental Capacity Act 2005 Code of Practice (Department for Constitutional Affairs 2007).

In *W v M* [2011] the Court of Protection concluded that, although each case must be considered individually, it is likely that for individuals in a VS the balance will probably fall towards withdrawing treatment. For clinically unstable individuals in an MCS, s(4) (Mental Capacity Act 2005) best interests will determine the lawfulness of withdrawing life-sustaining treatment in those particular circumstances. However, the position is clearer for people such as Mary: although they are in an MCS, they are otherwise in a clinically stable condition. For these people, withdrawal of treatment would never be in their best interests and would therefore be unlawful, and, with the necessary intent to kill, would be murder (*W v M* [2011] p1328).

More recently, in *Aintree University Hospitals NHS Foundation Trust v James* [2013], the Supreme Court confirmed that, whilst it will generally be in patients' best interests to act to preserve their life, it will not be in their best interests (Department for Constitutional Affairs 2007) to receive futile treatment. The Supreme Court disagreed that a proposed treatment should be regarded as futile if it offered no potential for cure or palliation, stating instead that a treatment will not be futile if it offers some benefit to the patient, even if it *has no effect upon the underlying disease or disability* (*Aintree University Hospitals NHS Foundation Trust v James* [2013] para 43).

Suicide and euthanasia

Until 1961 it was unlawful for someone to commit or attempt suicide, and until the Suicide Act 1961 was passed, anyone failing in an attempt to take his or her own life would face legal action. However, whilst it is no longer a crime to commit this act, it is still unlawful to assist a person who wants to bring his or her life to an end, and section 2 (1) Suicide Act 1961 makes the implications clear:

> *A person who aids, abets, counsels or procures the suicide of another, or an attempt by another to commit suicide, shall be liable on conviction on indictment to imprisonment for a term not exceeding fourteen years.*

Despite a number of recent cases (*Pretty v UK* [2002]; *Nicklinson, R. (on the application of) v Ministry of Justice* [2012]), there has been no shift in the legal position relating to assisted suicide, or euthanasia, as it is sometimes known. Whilst some commentators would argue that there is nothing ethically to distinguish between withdrawing or withholding treatments and acts deliberately intended to hasten someone's death, the law is very clear on the difference (*Airedale Hospital Trustees* v *Bland* [1993]) and it remains unlawful to commit such an act, regardless of the motives behind it.

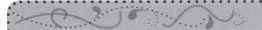

Chapter summary

This chapter has explored the law as it relates to some of the very difficult decisions that are made at the end of life. As the focus of care shifts from recovery to palliation many people are uncomfortable with the idea of either withdrawing or withholding active treatment; the sanctity of life is considered as part of this. We have explored the issue of consent and emphasised the importance of informed consent. Health care decisions at the end of life often involve a complex interplay of legal, ethical and professional issues that require careful consideration by the multidisciplinary team and may also even require a court declaration before care can continue. As a student health care professional you will find it very useful to understand the basis of these decisions, even if you disagree with them, but will not be expected (and indeed should not) make them on your own. Here are some useful summary points to support you to do this:

1. Health care professionals have a legal duty to provide care for their patients.
2. The standard of care will be judged against what is regarded (by other professionals) as acceptable at the time of treatment.
3. Patients have a right to refuse treatment or other therapeutic interventions.
4. Treatment without a patient's consent will usually be unlawful.
5. When a patient does not have the capacity to make decisions, there are legal guidelines that health care professionals should follow.
6. It may be lawful either to withdraw or withhold life-sustaining treatment.
7. It will never be lawful to end another person's life deliberately, or assist that person to take his or her own life.

Activities: brief outline answers

Activity 8.2: Decision making

Scenario 1

1. Does a duty of care exist? Yes, the neighbour principle in *Donoghue* v *Stevenson* [1932]. Martin could reasonably foresee that other people using the reception area could be affected by his acts or omissions. He therefore has a duty of care to them.
2. Has it been breached (either by doing something or failing to do something that a reasonable person would either have done or not done)? Would a 'reasonable person' (*Blyth* v *Birmingham Waterworks*

[1856]) throw a banana skin on to the floor? Probably not because a reasonable person would understand that there is a chance that someone could slip on it and suffer an injury.

3. Has harm been suffered? Yes – poor Simon broke his wrist as a direct result of slipping on the banana skin.
4. Of a type that is reasonably foreseeable? Yes – this type of injury is reasonably foreseeable.

There is therefore likely to be liability in negligence in this scenario.

Scenario 2

1. Does a duty of care exist? Yes, the neighbour principle in *Donoghue* v *Stevenson* [1932]. You should reasonably foresee that by leaving the gate open the cows might escape into the lane and therefore people using the lane, e.g. walkers, cyclists, motorists, could be affected by your omission. You therefore have a duty of care to them. You would also have a duty of care to the farmers as your failure to act is likely to affect them.
2. Has it been breached (either by doing something or failing to do something that a reasonable person would either have done or not done)? Would a 'reasonable person' (*Blyth* v *Birmingham Waterworks* [1856]) leave a gate in the countryside open? No – and it is also a breach of the countryside code.
3. Has harm been suffered? Yes – Emma has a fractured collar bone and her bike has been damaged. The farmer has suffered damage to livestock.
4. Of a type that is reasonably foreseeable? Yes – this type of injury/harm is reasonably foreseeable.

There is therefore likely to be liability in negligence in this scenario.

Further reading

Cooke, J. (2011) *Law of Tort*, 10th edn. Harlow: Pearson Education.

This text is written specifically for the student. It provides a clear explanation of the main principles of tort law.

Herring, J. (2010) *Medical Law and Ethics*. Oxford: Oxford University Press.

An overview of medical law as it relates to ethical theory and the current social and health care context.

Mason, J.K. and Laurie, G.T. (2013) *Law and Medical Ethics*, 9th edn. Oxford: Oxford University Press.

An overview of medical law and ethical theory within the context of contemporary health care. Recent developments in the law are also explored.

Slapper, G. and Kelly, D. (2013) *The English Legal System* 2013–2014, 14th edn. London: Routledge.

A critical exploration of the origins and development of English law, and how it is applied in practice.

Taylor, H. (2013) Determining capacity to consent to treatment. *Nursing Times*, 109 (43): 12–14.

This article provides further information about an individual's right to choose, the legal meaning of the word 'consent' and the importance of gaining consent before treating a patient.

Taylor, H. (2013) What does consent mean in clinical practice? *Nursing Times*, 109 (44): 30–32.

This article considers the meaning of consent in practice and explores the conditions that must be satisfied for consent to be valid.

Wheeler, H. (2012) *Law, Ethics and Professional Issues for Nursing*. London: Routledge.

Useful websites

http://www.gmc-uk.org/guidance/7046.asp

General Medical Council guidance on end of life care.

http://www.nmc-uk.org/Nurses-and-midwives/Regulation-in-practice/Regulation-in-Practice-Topics/consent

Nursing and Midwifery Council Regulations in Practice Guidance – Consent.

http://www.sii-mcpcil.org.uk/media/10843/LCP%20Core%20Documentation.pdf

Liverpool Care Pathway Core documentation.

References

Abernethy, A. and Wheeler, J.L. (2008) Total dyspnoea. *Current Opinion in Supportive and Palliative Care*, 2 (2): 110–113.

Adam, S.K. and Osborne, S. (2005) *Critical Care Nursing: Science and Practice*, 2nd edn. Oxford: Oxford University Press.

Aintree University Hospitals NHS Foundation Trust v *James* [2013] UKSC 67 (online). Available from: http://www.supremecourt.gov.uk/decided-cases/docs/UKSC_2013_0134_Judgment.pdf (accessed 12 November 2013).

Airedale Hospital Trustees v *Bland* [1992] UKHL 5 (4 February 1993) (online). Available from: http://www.bailii.org/uk/cases/UKHL/1992/5.html (accessed 19 July 2013).

Albert, N., Trochelman, K., Li, J. and Lin, S. (2010) Signs and symptoms of heart failure: are you asking the right questions? *American Journal of Critical Care*, 19 (5): 443–452.

Andershed, B. (2006) Relatives in end-of-life care – part 1: a systematic review of the literature the five last years, January 1999–February 2004. *Journal of Clinical Nursing*, 15: 1158–1169.

Aries, P. (1974) *Western Attitudes Towards Death: From the Middle Ages to the Present*. New York: Marion Boyars.

Astley-Pepper, M. (2005) Social erosion or isolation in palliative care. In: Nyatanga, B. and Astley-Pepper, M. (eds) *Hidden Aspects of Palliative Care*. London: Quay Books.

Barrett, D., Wilson, B. and Woollands, A. (2009) *Care Planning: A Guide for Nurses*. Harlow: Pearson Education.

Beauchamp, T. and Childress, J. (2009) *Principles of Biomedical Ethics*, 6th edn. Oxford: Oxford University Press.

Benjamin, M. and Curtis, J. (2010) *Ethics in Nursing: Cases, Principles and Reasoning*, 4th edn. Oxford: Oxford University Press.

Berry, J.W., Poortinga, Y.H., Segall, M.H. and Dasen, P.R. (1992) *Cross-cultural Psychology: Research and Applications*. Cambridge, MA: Cambridge University Press.

Bishop, A. and Scudder, J. (2001) *Nursing Ethics: Holistic Caring Practice*. Burlington, MA: Jones and Bartlett.

Blackman, N. (2008) The development of an assessment tool for the bereaved needs of people with learning disabilities. *British Journal of Learning Disability*, 36 (3): 165–170.

Blyth v *Birmingham Waterworks* [1856] 11 Exch 781 (online). Available from: Lexis®Library (accessed 21 July 2013).

Bolam v *Friern Management Committee* [1957] 2 All ER 118 (online). Available from: Lexis®Library (accessed 21 July 2013).

Bolitho v *City and Hackney H.A.* [1997] 4 All ER 771 HL (online). Available from: http://www.bailii.org/cgi-bin/markup.cgi?doc=/uk/cases/UKHL/1997/46.html&query=title+(+Bolitho+)&method=boolean (accessed 21 July 2013).

Brown, G. (2008) *The Living End: The Future of Death, Ageing and Immortality.* London: Macmillan.

Campinha-Bacote, J. (2002) The process of cultural competence in the delivery of healthcare services: a model of care. *Journal of Transcultural Nursing*, 13 (3): 181–184.

Campinha-Bacote, J. and Campinha-Bacote, D. (1999) A framework for providing culturally competent healthcare services in managed care organisations. *Journal of Transcultural Nursing*, 10 (4): 290–291.

Carlet, J., Thijs, L., Antonelli, M. *et al.* (2004) Challenges in end of life care in the ICU. Statement of the 5th International Consensus Conference in Critical Care: Brussels, Belgium, April 2003. *Intensive Care Medicine*, 30: 770–784.

Cassidy v *Ministry of Health* [1951] 1 All ER 574 (online). Available from: Lexis®Library (accessed 21 July 2013).

Chapman, L. (2009) Adapting the Liverpool Care Pathway for intensive care units. *European Journal of Palliative Care*, 16 (3): 116–118.

Cheraghi, M.A., Payne, S. and Mahvash, S. (2005) Spiritual aspects of end-of-life care for Muslim patients: experiences from Iran. *International Journal of Palliative Nursing*, 11 (9): 468–474.

Chester v *Afshar* [2004] UKHL 41 (online). Available from: http://www.bailii.org/cgi-bin/markup.cgi?doc=/uk/cases/UKHL/2004/41.html&query=title+(+chester+)+and+title+(+v+)+and+title+(+afshar+)&method=boolean (accessed 21 July 2013).

Chung, Y. (2000) Remembering spiritual care. *International Journal of Palliative Nursing*, 6 (9): 4.

Clarke, J. (2013) *Spiritual Care in Everyday Nursing Practice.* Basingstoke: Palgrave Macmillan.

Clements, P.T., Vigil, G.J., Manno, M.S. *et al.* (2003) Cultural perspectives of death, grief, and bereavement. *Journal of Psychosocial Nursing*, 41 (7): 18–26.

Cohen, S.L., Bewley, J.S., Ridley, S., Goldhill, D. and Members of The ICS Standards Committee (2003) Guidelines for the limitation of treatment for adults requiring intensive care. Intensive Care Society (online). Available from: http://www.ics.ac.uk/intensive_care_professional/standards_and_guidelines/limitation_of_treatment_2003 (accessed March 2011).

Collins v *Wilcock* [1984] 3 All ER 374 (online). Available from: Lexis®Library (accessed 21 July 2013).

Commissioning Board Chief Nursing Officer and DH Chief Nursing Adviser (2012) *Compassion in Practice: Nursing, Midwifery and Care Staff: Our Vision and Strategy.* NHS Commissioning Board (online). Available from: http://www.england.nhs.uk/wp-content/uploads/2012/12/compassion-in-practice.pdf (accessed 10 March 2014).

Coombs, M. and Long, T. (2008) Managing a good death in critical care: can health policy help? *Nursing in Critical Care*, 13 (4): 208–213.

Coombs, M.A., Addington-Hall, J. and Long-Sutehall, T. (2012) Challenges in transition from intervention to end of life care in intensive care: a qualitative study. *International Journal of Nursing Studies*, 49: 519–527.

Cortis, J. (2004) Meeting the needs of minority patients. *Journal of Advanced Nursing*, 48 (1): 51–58.

Covington, H. (2003) Caring presence: delineation of a concept for holistic nursing. *Journal of Holistic Nursing*, 21(3): 301–317.

Criminal Justice Act 1982 (c.48) (online). Available from: http://www.legislation.gov.uk/ukpga/1982/48/data.pdf (accessed 21 July 2013).

Criminal Justice Act 1988 (c.33) (online). Available from: http://www.legislation.gov.uk/ukpga/1988/33/data.pdf (accessed 21 July 2013).

Curtis, J.R. and Vincent, J. (2010) Ethics and end-of-life care for adults in the intensive care unit. *Lancet*, 376 (9749): 1347–1353.

De Souza, J. (2012) Calling in the palliative care team. In: Pettifer, A. and De Souza, J. (eds) *End-of-Life Nursing Care: A Guide for Best Practice*. London: SAGE.

Del Piccolo, L., Goss, C. and Zimmermann, C. (2006) Consensus finding on the appropriateness of provider responses to patient cues and concerns. *Journal of Patient Education and Counselling*, 61: 473–475.

Department for Constitutional Affairs (2007) *Mental Capacity Act 2005: Code of Practice*. London. The Stationery Office.

Department of Health (2000) *Comprehensive Critical Care: A Review of Adult Critical Care Services*. London: Department of Health.

Department of Health (2008) *End of Life Care Strategy: Promoting High Quality Care for All Adults at the End of Life*. London: Department of Health. Available from: www.dh.gov.uk/publications (accessed 29 June 2013)

Donoghue v *Stevenson* [1932] AC 562 (online). Available from: Lexis®Library (accessed 21 July 2013).

Eide, H., Quera, V., Graugaard, P. and Finset, A. (2004) Physician–patient dialogue surrounding patients' expression of concern: applying sequence analysis to RIAS. *Social Science and Medicine*, 59 (1): 145–155.

Ellis, H.K. and Narayanasamy, A. (2009) An investigation into the role of spirituality in nursing. *British Journal of Nursing*, 18 (14): 886–890.

Engebretson, J. (2002) Hands-on: the persistent metaphor in nursing. *Holistic Nursing Practice*, 16 (4): 20–35.

F v *West Berkshire Health Authority (Mental Health Act Commission intervening*) [1989] 2 All ER 545 (online). Available from: Lexis®Library (accessed 21 July 2013).

Fagan v *Metropolitan Police Commissioner* [1968] 3 All ER 442 (online). Available from: Lexis®Library (accessed 21 July 2013).

Family Law Reform Act 1969 (c.46) (online). Available from: http://www.legislation.gov.uk/ukpga/1969/46/data.pdf (accessed 21 July 2013).

Field, N.P. (2006) Unresolved grief and continuing bonds: an attachment perspective. *Death Studies,* 30: 739–756.

Firth, S. (2001) *Wider Horizons: Care of the Dying in a Multicultural Society.* London: National Council for Hospice and Specialist Palliative Care Services.

Francis, R. (2013) *Report of the Mid Staffordshire NHS Foundation Trust Public Inquiry.* London: The Stationery Office.

Freud, S. (1917) *Mourning and Melancholia. The Standard Edition of the Complete Psychological Works of Sigmund Freud, Volume XIV (1914–1916): On the History of the Psycho-Analytical Movement, Papers on Metapsychology and Other Works,* 237–258. London: Hogarth Press and Institute of Psycho-Analysis.

Gallagher, A. and Hodge, S. (2012) *Ethics, Law and Professional Issues: A Practice-Based Approach for Health Care Professionals,* 2nd edn. Hampshire: Palgrave MacMillan.

General Medical Council (2007) *0–18 Years: Guidance for All Doctors* (online). Available from: http://www.gmc-uk.org/static/documents/content/0–18-english-513_Revised.pdf (accessed 19 July 2013).

Gibbs, G. (1988) *Learning by Doing: A Guide to Teaching and Learning Methods.* Further Education Unit. Oxford: Oxford Polytechnic.

Gillick v *West Norfolk and Wisbech AHA* [1986] AC 112 (online). Available from: http://www.bailii.org/cgi-bin/markup.cgi?doc=/uk/cases/UKHL/1985/7.html&query=title+(+Gillick+)+and+title+(+v+)+and+title+(+West+)&method=boolean (accessed 19 July 2013).

Gold Standards Framework (2006) *Prognostic Indicator Paper vs 1.22.* England: Gold Standards Framework.

Goldberg, D.P., Jenkins, L., Millar, T. and Faragher, E.B. (1993) The ability of trainee general practitioners to identify psychosocial distress among their patients. *Psychological Medicine,* 23: 185–193.

Goodhead, A. (2010) A textual analysis of memorials written by bereaved individuals and families in a hospice context. *Mortality,* 15 (14): 323–339.

Gott, M., Seymour, J., Bellamy, G. and Ahmedzai, S. (2004) Older people's views about home as a place of care at the end of life. *Palliative Medicine,* 18: 460–467.

Govier, I. (2000) Spiritual care in nursing: a systematic approach. *Nursing Standard,* 14 (17): 32–36.

Greenstreet, W. (2004) Why nurses need to understand the principles of bereavement theory. *British Journal of Nursing,* 13 (10): 590–593.

Halsbury's Laws of England (2010a) *Negligence,* vol. 78, 5th edn (online). Available from: Lexis®Library (accessed 21 July 2013).

Halsbury's Laws of England (2010b) *Tort,* vol. 97, 5th edn (online). Available from: Lexis®Library (accessed 21 July 2013).

Halsbury's Laws of England (2011) *Medical Professions,* vol. 74, 5th edn (online). Available from: Lexis®Library (accessed 21 July 2013).

Hawley, G. (2007) *Ethics in Clinical Practice*. Edinburgh: Pearson.

Higginson, I.J. and Sen-Gupta, G.J.A. (2000) Place of care in advanced cancer: a qualitative systematic review of patient preferences. *Journal of Palliative Medicine*, 3: 287–300.

Humphrey, G.M. and Zimpfer, D.G. (2008) *Counselling for Grief and Bereavement*, 2nd edn. London: Sage Publications.

Huynh, T., Alderson, M., Thompson, M. *et al.* (2008) Emotional labour underlying caring: an evolutionary concept analysis. *Journal of Advanced Nursing*, 64 (2): 195–208.

Independent Review of the Liverpool Care Pathway (2013) *More Care, Less Pathway: A Review of the Liverpool Care Pathway* (online). Available from: https://www.gov.uk/government/uploads/system/uploads/attachment_data/file/212450/Liverpool_Care_Pathway.pdf (accessed 19 July 2013).

Intensive Care National Audit and Research Centre (2010) *CMP Case Mix and Outcome Summary Statistics* (online). Available from: https://www.icnarc.org/documents/summary%20statistics%20 2008–9.pdf (accessed 7 February 2014).

Intensive Care Society (2003) *Guidelines for Limitations of Treatment for Adults Requiring Intensive Care*. London: Intensive Care Society.

Intensive Care Society (2011) *End of Life Care for Adults* (online). Available from: http://www.nice.org.uk/guidance/qualitystandards/endoflifecare/home.jsp (accessed 26 January 2012).

James, N. (1989) Emotional labour: skill and work in the social regulation of feelings. *Sociological Review*, 37 (1): 15–42.

Kabat Zinn, J. (2011) *Mindfulness for Beginners*. Colorado: Boulder Press.

Kai, J., Bevan, J., Faull, C., Dodson, L., Paramjit, G. and Beighton, A. (2007) Professional uncertainty and disempowerment responding to ethnic diversity in healthcare: a qualitative study. *PLoS Medicine*, 4 (11): e323.

Klass, D., Silverman, P.R. and Nickman, S.L. (1996) *Continuing Bonds: A New Understanding of Grief*. Washington: Taylor Francis.

Kübler-Ross, E. (1973) *On Death and Dying*. London: Routledge.

Kwan, C.W.M. (2002) Families' experiences of the last office of deceased family members in the hospice setting. *International Journal of Palliative Nursing*, 8 (6): 266–275.

Levine, M.E. (1971) Holistic nursing. *Nursing Clinics of North America*, 6 (2): 253–264.

Lunney, J.R., Lynn, J. and Hogan, C. (2002) Profiles of older Medicare decedents. *Journal of the American Geriatric Society*, 50 (6): 1108–1112.

MacHale, R. and Carey, S. (2002) An investigation of the effects of bereavement on mental health and challenging behaviour in adults with learning disability. *British Journal of Learning Disabilities*, 30: 113–117.

Maciejewski, P.K., Zhang, B., Block, S.D. and Prigerson, H.G. (2007) An empirical examination of the stage theory of grief. *Journal of the American Medical Association*, 297 (7): 716–723.

Maguire, P., Faulkner, A., Booth, K., Elliot, C. and Hillier, V.F. (1996) Helping cancer patients disclose their concerns. *European Journal of Cancer*, 32: 78–81.

Maher, D. and Hemming, L. (2005) Understanding patient and family: holistic assessment in palliative care. *British Journal of Community Nursing*, 10 (7): 318–322.

Matsumoto, D. and Juang, L. (2007) *Culture and Psychology*. London: Wadsworth Publishers.

Matzo, M., Sherman, D., Lo, K., Egan, K., Grant, M. and Rhome, A. (2003) Strategies for teaching loss, grief and bereavement. *Nurse Educator*, 28 (2): 71–76.

McAree, S.J. and Doherty, P.A. (2010) A survey regarding physician preferences in end-of-life practices in intensive care across Scotland. *Journal of the Intensive Care Society*, 11 (3): 182–185.

McCallum, A. and McConigley, R. (2013) Nurses' perceptions of caring for dying patients in an open critical care unit: a descriptive exploratory study. *International Journal of Palliative Nursing*, 19 (1): 25–30.

McEvoy, L. and Duffy, A. (2008) Holistic practice: a concept analysis. *Nurse Education in Practice*, 8 (16): 412–419.

McGee, P. and Johnson, M.R.D. (2007) Developing culturally competent services in palliative care: management perspectives. In: Gatrad, R., Brown, E. and Sheikh, A. (eds) *Palliative Care for South Asians: Muslims, Hindus and Sikhs*. London: Quay Books.

MCPCIL (2011) Version 12 LCP-ICU LCP –ICU template (online). Available from: http://www. liv.ac.uk/media/livacuk/mcpcil/migrated-files/liverpool-care-pathway/updatedlcppdfs/LCP_ ICU_Version_12_Final_May_2011_EXAMPLE.pdf (accessed 10 March 2014).

McSherry, W. (2006) *Making Sense of Spirituality in Nursing and Health Care*, 2nd edn. London: Jessica Kingsley.

McSherry, W. and Jamieson, S. (2011) An online survey of nurses' perceptions of spirituality and spiritual care. *Journal of Clinical Nursing*, 20: 1757–1766.

Medical Research Council (2007) *Medical Research Council Dyspnoea Scale* (online). Available from: http://publications.nice.org.uk/chronic-obstructive-pulmonary-disease-cg101/ guidance#diagnosing-copd (accessed 14 March 2014).

Mehrabian, A. (1967) Significance of posture and position in the communication of attitude and status relationships. *Psychological Bulletin*, 71 (5): 359–372.

Mental Capacity Act 2005 (c.9) (online). Available from: http://www.legislation.gov.uk/ ukpga/2005/9/data.pdf (accessed 21 July 2013).

Molter, N.C. (1979) Needs of relatives of critically ill patients: a descriptive study. *Heart and Lung*, 8 (2): 332–339.

Mosby's Medical Dictionary (2009), 8th edn. St Louis: Elsevier.

Murray, S.A. and Sheikh, A. (2008) Care for all at the end of life. *British Medical Journal*, 336 (7650): 958–959.

National Council for Palliative Care (NCPC) (2012) *Dying Matters* (online). Available from: www. dyingmatters.org (accessed 6 February 2014).

National End of Life Care Programme (2010) *Holistic Common Assessment of Supportive and Palliative Care Needs for Adults Requiring End of Life Care*. National End of Life Care Programme (online). Available from: http://www.trinityhospice.co.uk/wp-content/uploads/2011/08/

l_-NHS_EoLC_Programme_Holistic_Common_Assessment_Document_2010.pdf (accessed 10 March 2014).

National Institute for Clinical Excellence (2004) *Improving Supportive and Palliative Care for Adults with Cancer: The Manual.* London: NICE.

National Institute for Clinical Excellence (2009) *Depression: The Treatment and Management of Depression in Adults.* London: NICE.

National Institute for Health and Clinical Excellence (2011) *End of Life Care for Adults Quality Standard* (online). Available from: http://publications.nice.org.uk/quality-standard-for-end-of-life-care-for-adults-qs13 (accessed 10 March 2014).

NHS Trust v *S* [2003] EWHC 365 (Fam) (online). Available from: http://www.bailii.org/cgi-bin/markup.cgi?doc=/ew/cases/EWHC/Fam/2003/365.html&query=title+(+NHS+)+and+title+(+Trust+)+and+title+(+v+)+and+title+(+S+)&method=boolean (accessed 19 July 2013).

Nicklinson, R. (on the application of) v *Ministry of Justice* [2012] EWHC 2381 (Admin) (online). Available from: http://www.bailii.org/cgi-bin/markup.cgi?doc=/ew/cases/EWHC/Admin/2012/2381.html&query=Nicklinson&method=boolean (accessed 21 July 2013).

Nicol, J. (2011) *Nursing Adults with Long Term Conditions.* Exeter: Learning Matters.

Nouwen, H.J. (1982) *In Memoriam.* Indiana: Ave Maria Press.

Nursing and Midwifery Council (2008) *The Code: Standards of Conduct, Performance and Ethics for Nurses and Midwives.* London: Nursing and Midwifery Council.

Nursing and Midwifery Council (2010) *Standards for Pre-registration Nursing Education.* London: Nursing and Midwifery Council.

Nyatanga, B. (2005) The concept of suffering: a hidden phenomenon. In: Nyatanga, B. and Astley-Pepper, M. (eds) *Hidden Aspects of Palliative Care.* London: Quay Books.

Nyatanga, B. (2008a) *Why Is It So Difficult to Die?* London: Quay Books.

Nyatanga, B. (2008b) Cultural competence: a noble idea in a changing world. *International Journal of Palliative Nursing,* 14 (7): 315.

Nyatanga, B. (2011) The pursuit of cultural competence: service accessibility and acceptability. *International Journal of Palliative Nursing,* 17 (5): 212–215.

Nyatanga, B. (2013) Attitudes to death: a time to pose difficult questions. *British Journal of Community Nursing,* 18 (10): 512.

Nyatanga, B. and de Vocht, H. (2009) When last offices are more than just a white sheet. *British Journal of Nursing,* 18 (17): 1028.

Nyatanga, L. and Nyatanga, B. (2011) Death and dying. In Birchenall, P. and Adam, N. (eds) *The Nursing Companion.* Basingstoke, Hampshire: Palgrave Macmillan.

Oberle, K. and Hughes, D. (2001) Doctors' and nurses' perceptions of ethical problems in end-of-life decisions. *Journal of Advanced Nursing,* 33 (6): 707–715.

Office for National Statistics (2011) *UK Census 2011* (online). Available from: http://www.ons.gov.uk/ons/guide-method/census/2011/census-data/index.html (accessed 6 February 2014).

O'Lynn, C. and Krautscheid, L. (2011) 'How should I touch you?': A qualitative study of attitudes on intimate touch in nursing care. *Advanced Journal of Nursing*, 111 (3): 24–31.

Parekh Report (2000) *The Future of Multi-Ethnic Britain*. London: Profile Books.

Pattison, N. (2008) Caring for patients after death. *Nursing Standard*, 22 (51): 48–56.

Pattison, N., Carr, S.M., Turnock, C. and Dolan, S. (2013) 'Viewing in slow motion': patients', families', nurses' and doctors' perspectives on end-of-life care in critical care. *Journal of Clinical Nursing*, 22: 1442–1454.

Payne, S. (2004) Loss and bereavement: overview. Cited in: Payne, S., Seymour, J. and Ingleton, C. (2004) *Palliative Care Nursing: Principles and Evidence for Practice*. Maidenhead: Open University Press.

Pretty v *UK* [2002] 35 EHRR 1 (online). Available from: http://www.bailii.org/cgi-bin/markup. cgi?doc=/eu/cases/ECHR/2002/427.html&query=pretty&method=boolean (accessed 21 July 2013).

Quested, B. and Rudge, T. (2003) Nursing care of dead bodies: a discursive analysis of last offices. *Journal of Advanced Nursing*, 41 (5): 553–560.

R (on the application of Burke) v *General Medical Council* [2005] All ER (D) 445 (online). Available from: Lexis®Library (accessed 8 August 2013).

R (Otley) v *Barking & Dagenham NHS PCT* [2007] EWCA Civ 392. http://www.bailii.org/ew/ cases/EWCA/Civ/2007/392.html (accessed 30 January 2014).

Radbruch, L. (2011) Foreword. In: Oliviere, D., Monroe, B. and Payne, S. (eds) *Death, Dying and Social Difference*. Oxford: Oxford University Press.

Re A (Medical Treatment: Male Sterilisation) [2000] 1 FCR 193 (online). Available from: Lexis®Library (accessed 21 July 2013).

Re MB (Medical Treatment) [1997] 2 FLR 426 (online). Available from: http://www.bailii.org/ cgi-bin/markup.cgi?doc=/ew/cases/EWCA/Civ/1997/3093.html&query=title+(+Re+)+and+title+ (+MB+)&method=boolean (accessed 19 July 2013).

Re T (An Adult: Refusal of Medical Treatment) [1992] 4 All ER 649 (online). Available from: Lexis®Library (accessed 21 July 2013).

Re W (A Minor) (Medical Treatment: Court's Jurisdiction) [1992] 4 All ER 627 (online). Available from: Lexis®Library (accessed 21 July 2013).

Read, S. (2006) *Palliative Care for People with Learning Disabilities*. London: Quay Books.

Rogers, M.E. (1970) *An Introduction to the Theoretical Base of Nursing*. Philadelphia, PA: FA Davis.

Ross, L. (1996) Teaching spiritual care to nurses. *Nurse Education Today*, 16: 38–43.

Saunders, C., Baines, M. and Dunlop, R. (1995) *Living with Dying: A Guide to Palliative Care*, 3rd edn. Oxford: Oxford Medical Handbooks.

Scholes, J. (2006) *Developing Expertise in Critical Care Nursing*. Chichester: Wiley/Blackwell.

Shannon, S.E., Long-Sutehall, T. and Coombs, M. (2011) Conversations in end of life care: communication tools for critical care practitioners. *Nursing in Critical Care*, 16 (3): 124–129.

Slapper, G. and Kelly, D. (2013) *The English Legal System* 2013–2014, 14th edn. London: Routledge.

Smart, F. (2005) The whole truth? *Nursing Management*, 11 (9): 17–19.

Stayt, L.C. (2009) Death, empathy and self-preservation: the emotional labour of caring for families of the critically ill in adult intensive care. *Journal of Clinical Nursing*, 18: 1267–1275.

Stroebe, M. and Schut, D. (1999) The dual process model of coping with bereavement: rationale and description. *Death Studies*, 23: 197–224.

Suicide Act 1961 (c. 60) (online). Available from: http://www.legislation.gov.uk/ukpga/Eliz2/9–10/60/data.pdf (accessed 19 February 2014).

Supply of Goods and Services Act 1982 (c.29) (online). Available from: http://www.legislation.gov.uk/ukpga/1982/29/data.pdf (accessed 21 July 2013).

Thomas, C. (2008) Dying: places and preferences. In: Payne, S., Seymour, J. and Ingleton, C. (eds) *Palliative Care Nursing: Principles and Evidence Based Practice*, 2nd edn. Maidenhead: McGraw-Hill, Open University Press.

Thomas, K. (2003) *Caring for the Dying at Home: Companions on the Journey*. Abingdon: Radcliffe Publishing.

Thompson, D.R., Hamilton, D.K., Cadenhead, C.D. *et al.* (2012) Guidelines for intensive care unit design. *Critical Care Medicine* 40 (5): 1586 (online). Available from: http://www.learnicu.org/SiteAssets/Pages/Guidelines/Guidelines%20for%20intensive%20care%20unit%20design.pdf (accessed 5 July 2013).

Tingle, J. and Cribb, A. (2007) *Nursing Law and Ethics*, 3rd edn. Oxford: Blackwell.

Tschudin, V. (eds) (2003) *Approaches to Ethics: Nursing Beyond Boundaries*. Boston: Harcourt.

Tuffrey-Wijne, I. and McEnhill, L. (2008) Communication difficulties and intellectual disability in end-of-life care. *International Journal of Palliative Nursing*, 14 (4): 189–194.

Twycross, R.G. (2003) *Introducing Palliative Care*, 4th edn. Oxford: Oxford University Press.

W (by her litigation friend B) v M (by her litigation friend the Official Solicitor) and others [2011] All Er 1313 (online). Available from: Lexis®Library (accessed 21 July 2013).

Walker, R. and Read, S. (2010) The Liverpool Care Pathway in intensive care: an exploratory study of doctor and nurse perceptions. *International Journal of Palliative Nursing*, 16 (6): 267–273.

Walsh, D. and Nelson, K. (2003) Communication of a cancer diagnosis: patients' perception of when they were first told they had cancer. *American Journal of Hospice and Palliative Care*, 20 (1): 52–56.

Walter, T. (1996) A new model of grief: bereavement and biography. *Mortality*, 1 (1): 7–25.

White, L., Duncan, G. and Baumle, W. (2010) *Foundations of Nursing*, 3rd edn. Michigan: Delmar.

Woodrow, P. (2011) *Intensive Care Nursing: A Framework for Practice*, 3rd edn. London: Routledge.

World Health Organization (1990) *Technical Report*, series 804. Geneva: World Health Organization.

World Health Organization (2012) *WHO Definition of Palliative Care*. Available at: www.who.int/cancer/palliative/definition/en (accessed 16 March 2013).

Zimmerman, C., Del Piccolo, L. and Mazzi, M.A. (2003) Patient cues and medical interviewing in general practice: examples of the application of sequential analysis. *Epidemiologia e Psichiatria Sociale*, 12 (2): 115–123.

Index